D0221490

NEXT PANDA, PLEASE!

Further Adventures of a Wildlife Vet

ALSO BY DAVID TAYLOR

Going Wild

Zoovet

Doctor in the Zoo

Next Panda, Please!

Further Adventures of a Wildlife Vet

DAVID TAYLOR

STEIN AND DAY / *Publishers* / New York

First published in the United States of America in 1983
Copyright ©1982 by David C. Taylor
All rights reserved
Printed in the United States of America

STEIN AND DAY / *Publishers*
Scarborough House
Briarcliff Manor, N.Y. 10510

Library of Congress Cataloging in Publication Data

Taylor, David, 1934-
    Next panda, please!

    1. Taylor, David, 1934-   2. Veterinarians—
England—Biography.   3. Wildlife diseases.
4. Zoo animals—Diseases.   I. Title.
SF613.T38A36   1982   636.089′092′4 [B]   81-48442
ISBN 0-8128-2857-7

This book is dedicated to
Jodie Elizabeth Greenwood and Jennifer Jane Nutkins
in the certainty that they will become animal people,
and to Martin Robert Massey who is already one.

1

'Do you like warthogs?' my hostess asked, as casually as other folk might ask about one's taste in music or how many sugars you take in your tea.

Up to that point I don't think I'd considered at any length whether I was pro- or anti-warthog. I'd once smashed up a car in northern Kenya by driving into a hole dug by a warthog: they have a habit of building such pitfalls. On the other hand, warthogs in zoos are generally very popular, affable creatures that adapt well and have gentle natures. Their comical faces attract the visitors and they give little trouble, being robust, easy to feed and long-lived. On the few occasions that I'd had to treat a warthog it had usually been for arthriticky joints brought on by advancing years. One dear old soul at Belle Vue Zoo, Manchester, had lived for 16½ years without a day's illness. Yes, very definitely, now that I came to think about it, I liked warthogs a lot. I have found them, like all members of the pig family, to be clean in their habits, intelligent and full of character.

'Yes,' I replied to the question, 'I like warthogs. Why?'

'There's a lovely warthog boar living in the bush not far away. Walter's his name. He absolutely adores potatoes. I'll go and fetch some and then we'll call him.'

My hostess was Betty Leslie-Melville, a remarkable lady who at her home in Kenya had raised a young giraffe, Daisy Rothschild, and returned her to the wild. Tame giraffes and now spuds as bait for a wild warthog! Betty Leslie-Melville certainly had a way with wildlife.

When she returned with a bag of potatoes, she told me to sit on the grass at the edge of the terrace with a small mound of the vegetables close to my feet. I was not to move or say anything. 'Walter is a bit on the nervous side,' she explained. Then she began calling towards the forest: 'Wal-ter! W-a-a-alter! Wa-a-a-a-alter!'

It was really rather exciting, sitting on the grass and waiting for the bush to yield up two hundredweights of untamed warthog with ferocious-looking curved tusks that may be over two feet in length. Tame as they may be in captivity, wild warthog boars can be dangerous, cantankerous individuals.

'Wa-a-a-a-lter!' Betty continued to call. 'He may perhaps be out of earshot, foraging with his band.'

Suddenly there was a warthog in the distance. Out of the woodland beyond the lawn he came, ears pricked and piggy tail curved high. He hesitated for a moment as he broke cover, stared in our direction and then began to trot towards us. Betty called his name one last time and then reminded me to stay still and silent.

Walter came on steadily. He was a magnificent individual, standing over two feet high with a pair of beady black eyes set in the knobbly, ferocious-looking face. His bristly head and bold and jaunty bearing reminded me strongly of a moustachioed and irascible sergeant-major. When he was ten yards from me the warthog stopped and eyed me intently. His tail was now held high in the air and the crest of straggly hair running down his back was partially raised. He sniffed, switched his gaze to the mound of potatoes and decided to risk a brush with the stranger. Ever so slowly he edged forwards, eyes darting up and down from me to the potatoes and back again. I could smell warthog now and I could see the cracks in the beauty mask of dried mud that covered his fierce face. I held my breath. It was a magical moment. No crush-cage, no tranquillisers, no ropes or bars or protective moats filled with water. Here was one of those rare occasions when, without the help of such artificial devices, one can meet up with a wild animal face to face. OK, so Walter was only a 'cupboard-love', out to free-load on the tasty potatoes, but even so, man as a rule is shunned by his fellow-creatures as a dangerous and untrustworthy species, and exceptions to the rule are very precious.

Walter arrived at my shoes. He was wary and wound-up like a coiled spring. He gobbled tensely at the potatoes, his front feet doing a sort of little teetering dance. so anxious were they to get him away from the strange-smelling ape as soon as his meal was finished. Very, very slowly I moved my right hand down my legs. Walter kept his eye on me but continued to eat. My hand was twelve inches, then six, then three away from his curly upper tusks. Breathlessly I pushed my hand forwards just a fraction more. I touched the hard ivory. Walter finished his meal, grunted quietly and backed off, but I had actually touched a wild, conscious warthog. As Walter wandered aimlessly back towards the forest, his portly belly replete and his tail switching back and forth, I knew that this was the high point of my visit to Kenya.

My encounter with Walter came some ten years after I'd decided to turn my back on my old life as a vet to every sort of domestic animal, and to concentrate only on the wild and exotic species. In that time I'd clocked up over a quarter of a million miles in aeroplanes, worked in thirty-one countries and spent around fifty thousand pounds in air fares. But life was far from being all champagne and oysters and cuddly koala bears (koala bears are by nature generally cantankerous and they bite and scratch at the drop of a hat). The life of a vagabond veterinarian, constantly on the move and denied even the generous periods of 'shore leave' enjoyed by seafarers, produces numerous difficulties. I was accustomed to being abroad on family birthdays and great festivals. I'd missed three Christmases and two New Years, broken innumerable dinner appointments, wasted theatre tickets and interrupted holidays with my wife, Shelagh, and my two daughters. All the same – and an element of selfishness is undeniable – I didn't regret a moment of it. The strange, wandering work was deep in my blood now and the days of dogs and cats, pigs and cattle seemed part of a previous incarnation. The idea of returning to general practice in my home town of Rochdale or à la Herriot was unimaginable. It still is.

Fate had played other cards also. During my travels in England I had met Hannelore Lonkwitz, an attractive German from East

Prussia and a friend of my sister. She lived near Windsor and began accompanying me first to the safari park there and then to the London Dolphinarium and further afield. Hanne and I became great friends. With Jim McNab, the Oliver Hardy-esque head keeper at Windsor, Hanne learned to shoot the dart-rifle with accuracy, using cardboard boxes as targets. The three of us spent many hours traipsing on foot around the lion and tiger reserves, unprotected from the big cats which were at the time immature and unlearned in the ways of stalking and harrying humans; that all stopped when one notable day a lion rushed the secretary of the Zoo Federation, who was making an official visit, and put him in hospital.

Hanne also helped me when I went sampling dolphins. In those years the South Coast was dotted with dolphin pools during the summer season. At the high point, around 1972, there had been twenty-two dolphinaria in England and Scotland. Hanne quickly learned the 'feel' of marine mammals, seeing beyond the perpetual smile of the bottle-nosed dolphin that will often feed and play right up to the point of death. Every few weeks we spent an evening at the London Dolphinarium in Oxford Street, doing health checks in the cramped conditions under Soho Square after the last show.

Examining a dolphin means hauling the animal out of the water. Few folk can catch a dolphin swimming free in deep water without the use of a soft net that is deep enough to reach the bottom and is well weighted with lead. Dolphins rather enjoy the business of being caught for medical examinations, I suspect; if you are a dolphin there is plenty of opportunity for play and for making fools of the humans handling the netting. There are so many delightful variations of the catching game. There is, for example, the jump over the net. This ploy can be followed by lifting the bottom of the net or by squeezing between the edge of the net and the wall. Or you may elect to swim straight into the net underwater, feign unconsciousness and then, when the panicking homo sapiens struggle to pull you up or – super wheeze – order a fully-clothed fellow to jump in to your assistance, you pull your snout out of the net, slip over it into clear water and give all those on shore a thorough dowsing with one flick of your tail.

4

Should some bloke fancy his chances of grabbing you when the net slowly approaches and he bobs in the water with his mask, snorkel and flippers, ready to pounce next time you come up to breathe, it is rather a lark deftly to snatch off his snorkel or relieve him of a rubber flipper. Humans, you have observed, are about as competent in your environment as the lumps of waterlogged driftwood you remember from your days off the Florida Keys. What really screws the landlubbers up, though, is the one about lying on the bottom of the pool for minutes and minutes on end. They're up there waiting for you to surface. As time goes by they become impatient and anxious, and forget the scientific fact that dolphins can hold their breaths for about seven times as long as humans. Sure enough, eventually they'll send down some awkward individual to see what's up; then you nip him on the kneecap and in the confusion as he scuttles back to shore you escape. After each successful escape, of course, you stick your head perkily out of the water, chatter impudently and ask for a fish reward.

Dolphin games like this may seem an infuriating waste of time to the human beings involved, but they once saved my life. I had arranged to blood-sample some dolphins at a Majorca marineland and then go straight to the airport to travel back to London in the company of the wife of one of the marineland's directors. So well did the dolphins play their game that I suggested that the lady should go on ahead to check in and I would join her at the last minute just as soon as these so-and-so animals decided to stop fooling around and let me take the miserable teaspoonful of blood that I required. We struggled to catch the beasts but relentlessly, and with blatant sparkles in their wide, black eyes, they gave us a very hard time. Everyone except the dolphins became irritable and when at last I obtained my samples I found that I had missed my plane; the next flight was on the following day and there was a sick Père David's deer to see at the zoo in Manchester. So it was in a distinctly niggly mood that I was walking out of the marineland to check in again at the hotel I had left that morning, when I met the company's public relations man coming in the opposite direction. On seeing me he acted in a peculiar fashion. He suddenly sat down on the dusty ground, went white as a bottle of penicillin, pointed one arm and long finger at me and croaked, 'You're dead!'

He was on his way back from Santanyi airport with terrible news: the Iberia plane on which I'd been booked had collided in the air with a Spantax charter near the French border. Everyone on the Iberia aircraft had perished, including the director's wife, and my name was on the list of boarding passengers. A miss may perhaps be as good as a mile, but both the PR man, who had known nothing about my delay caused by the bolshie dolphins, and I needed several large Carlos Primero coñacs to recover. Ever since, I have discovered wells of unlimited patience when waiting for dolphin patients to be nabbed and presented for examination.

Hanne was with me on the night at the London Dolphinarium when I was faced with the problem of an old dolphin on whom I was finding it impossible to locate a blood vessel for sampling. Terry Nutkins, the friend in charge of the day-to-day welfare of the animals, and other experienced dolphin handlers crowded around as I fumbled and fumed. There wasn't a sign of the dark shadow or faint groove denoting the uniquely designed heat-exchange veins of the animal. Advice was proffered, folk puffed and blew and the director became increasingly impatient. Embarrassing failure.

Then Hanne, who was holding my sample bottles and sticky labels, leaned over the top of the crouching men's heads, stuck out an elegant finger at an invisible point on the grey tail-fluke and said in ringing tones, 'Entschuldigung, excuse me. Put the needle there.' The men, myself included, chuckled patronisingly. Who had ever heard of a blood vessel lying so far from the fluke edge? Dolphin anatomy is consistent and unvarying. 'There!' Hanne repeated. Oh these Prussians, I thought silently, but I stuck the needle in where she'd indicated. One more failure to strike oil wouldn't hurt. Immediately a healthy stream of blood began to fill my sample tube. Hanne's reputation as a diviner of difficult dolphins was instantly established and she ceased to be regarded as just the 'bit of fluff' that I frequently had in tow.

It was perhaps inevitable that Hanne and I should fall in love as I felt my ties with the North, with the stony moors and drizzly streets of Lancashire – even with Shelagh – loosening. I had begun to think about the previously unthinkable: of starting a new life away from the old farmhouse on the edge of the town where I had been born, away from the warm and open vitality of the old cotton-town lifestyle with its temper as resilient and unpretentious as a steaming plate of tripe and onions, and its cutting edge as sharp as the wind that sweeps down the flanks of the Pennines, chivvying the blackened stone farmhouses and the grime-grey nomadic bands of Lonk sheep.

In due course Hanne and I both became divorced, and together we bought a little house in Lightwater in Surrey in which to set up a new home with Hanne's two sons, Andreas and Martin. The once unthinkable split from Lancashire had happened, but I still travelled north regularly to keep in touch with things at Belle Vue, the zoo in Manchester where I was responsible for the veterinary care of the animals, and to visit the practice's northern office at the Keighley home of my partner, Andrew Greenwood.

Meanwhile out home in Lightwater became the southern office, so Hanne would hold the fort whenever I was away and I would telephone her regularly. While I was visiting Betty Leslie-Melville in Kenya I phoned home and Hanne gave me some wonderful news. Dr Marguerita Celma, biological director of Madrid Zoo, had rung to say that they were going to receive a pair of giant pandas.

'Ask the Royal College library to get me photocopies of everything that has been published on pandas,' I told Hanne, literally tingling with excitement. 'Can you imagine what this means to me? Something I never dared dream about. Handling a giant panda.'

'You're surely not hoping they'll fall ill, I trust,' she said reprovingly.

'Of course not. But I want to touch one.'

I'd seen almost all the pandas then in captivity in China during a visit to that country in 1974, and I'd seen the London, Washington and Paris animals on several occasions, but I'd never come anywhere near touching, let alone getting involved in the care and treatment

7

of, these mysterious creatures. The Chinese officials who had showed my companion, Gary Smart, and me round the panda pavilions of Peking, Canton and Shanghai had been ultra-cautious in making sure that we stood well away from bars or mesh separating us from the animals. The way our hosts had hovered round us, gripped our arms and flung themselves in front of us whenever we made to move a little closer might well have given the impression that either we were blundering imbeciles or the pandas were the meanest things on four legs since tyrannosaurus rex.

'Do you think they're frightened we might try to assassinate the beasts?' Gary had whispered to me on one occasion when we had tried doubling back into the service area behind Peking's panda installation to see what would happen if we approached the apparently easy-going, bamboo-scrunching pandas without a wall of nervous, blue-kapok-clad Chinese around us. It hadn't worked. The human wall had eyes in the back of their heads, had tumbled to what we were about and had doubled back even more nippily than ourselves. In everyone's haste some of the footwork wasn't too fancy, our interpreter had tripped, bringing me crashing down as well, and the entire official party had ended up in a tangled heap in front of the pandas who had diplomatically pretended not to notice. Gary and I had been given a few hairy words of comradely correction and, I'm sure as a punishment, taken to the theatre that evening to see the same knee-achingly tedious performance of *The White-haired Girl*, a revolutionary opera that we'd been obliged to sit through the night before!

Not that I have ever had any illusions about pandas being cuddly teddy-bears. Although not bears, giant pandas have the weight, compactness and powerful bite of a bear the size of, say, the Himalayan black. Such a creature can easily mangle a man if it has a mind to, and as well as bear-like claws that can rake savagely, there is that special steely 'thumb', the inside digit of the fore-feet, that has been specially adapted for grasping cane. If one of those latched onto your more tender parts in anger, it would make the iron hand of 'Jaws' in the James Bond movies seem as delicate as a geisha girl's by comparison. And pandas, natural loners who haunt the dense bamboo forests that cling to the high mountain slopes of remote Szechuan, are not surprisingly enigmatic and difficult to understand. Their temperament can be mercurial and unpredictable and some, particularly as they grow older, become quite savage.

No, I wasn't foolhardy enough to think that I could rush up to a panda as it lay on its back, drooling over the thick stem of sugar-cane that it was feeding into its mouth with both hands, and tickle its tummy button. I just wanted to be involved, to have the opportunity somehow to work on a giant panda. My only chance was for pandas to arrive at one of the zoos where I worked, which in the past had seemed an impossible dream: the few specimens released by the Chinese were sent to the capital-city zoos of friendly nations. London has its pair − but its own in-house veterinary institute as well. I had had to make do with studying and occasionally treating the lovely lesser panda, a very different animal.

Now it had happened. Mao was dead and China was looking for friends. Franco was dead and Spain under King Juan Carlos was also adopting a new outward-looking style. What the global social and political implications of thes' sea-changes might be is the stuff that statesmen ponder. The little plum that fell off the tree as far as I was concerned was the gift which the Chinese gave to His Hispanic Majesty. Where President Brezhnev is said to have a garage full of luxurious foreign automobiles that have been presented to him, and ex-President Giscard d'Estaing was in the habit of coming back from State visits to Central Africa with his pockets full of sparklers, King Juan Carlos, like Ted Heath before him, had collared a couple of the most fabulous of rare mammals. However, he couldn't quite see the pandas doing their business all over the thick blue carpets of the Palacio Real, so he farmed out his two priceless presents to a new zoo barely a mile from His Majesty's bathroom window, a zoo where I was already working regularly as veterinary consultant.

The Madrid Zoo is one of the loveliest parks in Europe. Set in the extensive Casa de Campo woodland just outside the city centre, it is brilliantly designed to provide an environment which is attractive to visitors but at the same time good for the animals to live in. Rather than re-working old naturalistic ideas of zoo design by trying to reproduce, often impossibly, little bits of appropriate habitat, the zoo uses modern concrete architecture and good gardening to give the animals something functionally and psychologically fulfilling. Although patently artificial, it is also very easy on the eye of the human visitor. For example, instead of clambering over fake mini-mountains of gunnite, the ibexes have a great concrete 'wedding-cake', the work of one of Spain's leading sculptors. It doesn't pretend to be a mountain but it gives the species for which it was designed an exciting and harmonious environment on which to play battle, spy out the land or doze peacefully in the hot midday. The zoo possesses an extensive collection including such important creatures as okapi, giant South American otters, Imperial eagles and Atlas Mountain lions; those are names to conjure with!

When I arrived at Heathrow from Nairobi, Hanne picked me up in the car, as she always does after anything but the briefest trip abroad, and handed me a couple of photographs. 'Arrived this morning from Madrid,' she said. They were shots of the two new giant pandas, 'Chang-Chang' and 'Shao-Shao', being unloaded at Barajas airport under the watchful eye of my good friend, Antonio-Luis, curator and assistant veterinarian at Madrid's Zoo de la Casa de Campo.

As soon as we reached the house I booked two seats on the first flight to Madrid next day, and we arrived at the zoo in typically bitter cold winter weather. I like the stillness of the park under the eggshell-blue sky at that time of year. The animals seem more relaxed then. There is an air of subdued expectancy as everyone waits for the first sign of spring. Many females are heavy with young. The sounds of the zoo, the soft whoopings, clicks, shufflings and throaty rumblings travel more clearly through the frosty air. The buffaloes and the elephant seals blow lazy puffs of smoke as they stick their heads out of doors and sniff to see what is in the wind. Best of all there are few visitors around, no children yelling, no aroma of perspiring pram-pushers and chocolate milk.

We walked straight from the taxi to the new panda house. Antonio-Luis and his wife, Liliana, an attractive Argentinian lady who is chief veterinarian of the zoo and a close friend of ours, were

10

there, supervising the preparation of the pandas' lunch by the full-time panda staff — a biologist and two senior keepers, all in white uniforms, whose only job was to take care of the two new arrivals. Pandas always command a substantial retinue, even more so than dolphins and whales, and the Mexican pandas actually have their own veterinarian who practises on nothing else but them (not a good idea, in my opinion).

Proud as new parents, Antonio-Luis and Liliana introduced us to Chang-Chang and Shao-Shao. There they were, with their individual comfortable sleeping quarters and grassy paddock as well as the attached keepers' room (including a bed, for the animals were being tended round the clock), kitchen and crush-cage. This latter had been built as part of a passageway that they would use routinely every day and it incorporated a remotely controlled weighing-machine.

The pandas were magnificent animals, obviously in spanking condition and with hearty appetites. They relished the Spanish bamboo and smacked their lips over the fresh-cooked rice and cereal balls garnished with grated carrot and apple. To my utter delight I was actually able to go into the quarters of the male, Chang-Chang, and, while giving him a bowl of warm milk, reach out with the other hand and gently touch him. I felt the hair — coarser and more greasy than I had imagined — and prodded the stocky body: fantastic! Chang-Chang regarded me blandly with eyes like beads of black oil and didn't utter a sound. It wasn't thought advisable to take the same liberties with Shao-Shao, who was claimed by the Chinese to be a 'test-tube baby', produced by artificial insemination, and was considered to be a much more tetchy individual. Hanne, however, seemed to get on great guns with her through the feeding-trap in her door by blowing up her nostrils à la Barbara Woodhouse.

The zoo had pulled out all the stops in trying to provide happy and healthy conditions for the two animals. There was heating for winter and a shady porch and water-shower for the summer; I wondered whether they would be enough to keep the pandas cool during the baking-hot days of July and August. Perhaps air-conditioning might be necessary, since giant pandas with their thick fur coats don't like too much heat.

We discussed the diet. Fresh bamboo from what we hoped were unpolluted parts of the countryside would arrive daily and be stored in a cool room. Before feeding, just to be extra-careful in case some careless farmer had let insecticide sprays drift onto the bamboo, it was all to be thoroughly washed in clean water.

At the time there was precious little material published on the biology and care of the species but what there was I'd read, and I'd talked or corresponded with the few veterinarians worldwide who had experience of pandas. One immediate decision that I had to take was what preventive medicine measures to institute, if any. I collected a dropping sample to take home for parasite examination, as I wasn't keen on administering worming medicines to an 'unknown' kind of animal if they weren't necessary. Protection against virus diseases was a prime consideration, but what sorts of virus might go for giant pandas? More importantly, what would the effect of vaccines against some of those viruses be on these strange beasts? A vaccine that is well-tolerated and free of side-effects in one species can sometimes induce unpleasant, dangerous or even fatal results in some other sort of animal. I'd known sheep and pig vaccines cause big trouble in dolphins, while domestic cat vaccines were frequently risky in cheetahs and smaller exotic cats. And of course no pharmaceutical company produces any sort of vaccine specially for our friend *Ailuropoda melanoleuca*, the giant panda.

Antonio-Luis asked me how I would make my decision on vaccination. After some thought I told him that it would seem sensible to innoculate Chang-Chang and Shao-Shao against diseases known to threaten the pandas' closest relatives. Pandas belong to a zoological family called the Procyonidae. The family embraces the raccoons, coatis and kinkajous, as well as a couple of creatures that most folk have never even heard of: the cacomistle and the very rarely exhibited alingo. The procyonids can be affected by the common feline enteritis virus (although they don't seem to suffer from cat 'flu) and like many zoos, Madrid acts as a magnet to the local moggies who come a-foraging. Nor can Rentokil in all its glory eliminate the sizeable rodent population found in every zoo and the attendant risk of rat- or mouse-borne infections such as leptospirosis, a bacterial disease. It was very unlikely that my new charges would come into contact with any dogs, even though the panda's procyonid cousins are open to dog distemper and hepatitis viruses and, like all animals, to the deadly rabies bug. Also, no killed distemper vaccines were being produced any longer and I wanted to use killed rather than live vaccines to minimise the risk of reaction. I would also use good old British products made by firms I trusted. This wasn't mere chauvinism; my partner, Andrew Greenwood, had cultured dangerous bacteria from many unopened bottles of so-called killed vaccines manufactured in Europe.

The risk of rabies was infinitesimally small, as the disease was not present in the Madrid region although it did lurk in the wildlife in some areas of Spain. I made my decision. We would give the pandas killed feline enteritis vaccine and also protect them against leptospirosis. I suggested to Liliana and Antonio-Luis that we put the animals into the crush-cage and got the inoculation done straightaway.

It was obvious that my friends were more than a little apprehensive. Their faces dropped. Were we going to upset the apple cart by interfering? Wouldn't it be better to let sleeping dogs lie? I could read it on their faces although no-one said anything.

'Don't worry,' I said. 'There's no sense in waiting. If we're going to do it at all, the sooner the better. I guarantee there will be no side-effects.' For someone about to jab a needle into his first giant panda I must have sounded outrageously rash.

'If there is a reaction, how soon after the injection might it occur?' Hanne's voice sounded slightly diffident.

'Oh, long before our flight is due to leave for London, darling,' I replied. 'There'll be plenty of time for the Guardia Civil to close the borders!' I laughed a small hollow laugh; dammit, any more of this and they would start giving me real doubts.

Liliana and Antonio-Luis at least knew exactly the importance of protection by vaccination. Sometimes non-veterinary folk in positions of power in a zoo seem to think that preventive medicine is tempting fate and a waste of money, even in these enlightened days of regular medical check-ups and compulsory vaccination for human beings. At an English safari park where I'd instructed vitamin E to be mixed daily with the giraffe food ever since some sudden deaths years earlier due to a deficiency that damaged heart muscle, I was astonished to be called to another dead animal that showed the typical post-mortem features of the lack of vitamin E. It didn't take me long to discover that a director had ordered the vitamin supplement to be stopped as 'an expensive luxury'. 'After all,' he had said to the curator as he justified his order, 'the giraffes are fit as fleas and breeding well. Why give medicine?' It was as a newly-qualified young vet working on the Pennine farms round Rochdale that I'd first met this sort of attitude. A shepherd had sustained heavy losses each spring in his young lambs. Investigation had shown the cause to be an infectious complaint commonly called pulpy kidney disease, and I had got the shepherd to inject his flock each year with a cheap, effective vaccine. The results, as expected, had been dramatic: not a lamb lost from pulpy kidney during the lambing season. Then, after three years, the shepherd had complained to me about the losses starting again, and he was as puzzled as I was when I found classical pulpy kidney at post-mortem. After I had questioned him, however, the explanation was revealed. He had stopped vaccination. 'Why did you do that,' I had asked, 'when your results had been so spectacular?' His answer had been defiantly forthright: 'Nay, Doctor, dawn't tha see? There weren't no trouble in t' sheep. Naw sense i' physickin' t' buggers if'n there's nowt up wi' 'em.'

As far as I could see there was 'nowt up' with the pandas as we enticed first one and then the other into the crush-cage with apples. Once an animal was in, Antonio-Luis gently slid the barred sides of the cage inwards and when the panda was firmly squeezed, locked them in position. That was when we first witnessed the remarkable agility of the animal. We knew that pandas are naturally far better tree-climbers than bears but now, compressed into a space no bigger than itself, the panda performed acrobatics more effortlessly than

14

any monkey. They were both the same, able to stand on their heads or twirl through 360 degrees as if the steel bars were made of india-rubber. To do a confined head-stand, Chang-Chang simply stuck his head into his springy belly and with a powerful flick of his wrists turned himself over. The curious thing was the silence of their performances. Where monkeys in similar situations would holler and scold and bears would growl threats, the pandas went through their routine of making their buttocks an impossible moving target for my needle without making a murmur. There was no sign of agitation or apprehension, just cool, practical bloody-mindedness. So don't be misled by his portly figure and plodding gait — for my money, the giant panda must be acclaimed the con-tortionist extraordinaire of the zoo world. I suppose you get good at such things if you live in impenetrable bamboo forest.

Eventually, after being made to look the most un-dextrous of fools, I was able to give the vaccines. The prick of the needle produced no show of anger or irritation. Released from the crush-cage, the pandas retired tranquilly to their quarters to sample armfuls of leafy bamboo. Nor did they show any signs of delayed reaction to the vaccination, I was relieved to find, and the next day we returned home. As I sat on the plane I wondered when I might have another chance to handle the pandas. What would I be faced with if one fell ill?

My next case, however, concerned a very different creature, a peace-loving, nocturnal, armour-plated character from South America. Armadillos aren't found naturally in Europe, still less in Great Britain, and as for London's Notting Hill Gate — you'd find a more likely armadillo stamping-ground on the moon. Yet here, one wet Saturday night, a small six-banded armadillo was to be found curling itself into a miserable ball beside some rubbish bins at the back of a pub. There was no hospitable brown pampas earth to dig into for shelter anywhere around. At around nine o'clock a group of teenage boys, pausing to light cigarettes and relieve themselves against a wall, stumbled across what they took to be this 'balding hedgehog' of considerable size — about as big as a football. As townies, they may well have never seen a real live hedgehog. Guffawing, they gathered round the curious creature. A tentative prod with a toe-cap provoked a tighter in-rolling of the 'hedgehog'; it was alive!

I suppose that while the lads were as familiar as the next Londoner with the sort of things to be found behind public houses, a hedgehog (or armadillo) wasn't one of them. In their eyes, the natural thing to do to any piece of wayside bric-à-brac like tin cans, empty cartons and chunks of brick – even bald hedgehogs that insisted on masquerading as footballs – was to kick it. So that's what they did to the armadillo. It wasn't an easy thing to propel with your foot. There was no chance of lofting it into the air, but you could just about dribble it round the corner and onto the pavement. Maybe it would roll easier on the flagstones.

The youths shouted and crowed as they got into the feel of the game and reached the street. But it did make your foot ache, punting it along. One of the party braced himself over the grey trembling ball and prepared his shot. His wet boot gleamed in the light of a street lamp as it travelled through the air. It was a good kick by any standards, with the right use of the instep and the full force of the thigh muscles behind it – they'd seen no better at Spurs' ground that afternoon – and it produced an audible grunt from the armadillo as it thudded into the animal's chest. It also smashed one of the bones of the foreleg.

Whatever Incan or Aztec god watches over armadillos intervened at that point in the one-sided game, in the shape of two doughty old ladies hurrying home bent behind umbrellas. The pair stepped into a shop doorway as the hooting band of youths came towards them. 'They're kicking something along, Alice,' said one. She peered through rain-spattered spectacles into the gloomy street. Her companion tut-tutted and craned her neck to look. 'Wait a minute, wait a minute, it's a *cat*!'

There was a second's pause before the two women launched themselves, umbrellas cleaving the air and voices strident with outrage, at the startled boys. Old ladies have frequently been 'gone over' by such valiant troops of marauders, but on this occasion the youths mouthed a few ripe obscenities, shrugged their dampening shoulders and marched off into the night. The hedgehog hadn't been much of a ball anyway. Leave it to the loony old bags then, for Chrissake.

'Wicked, wicked people in the world!' seethed Alice as she bent to pick up the apparently lifeless moggy. Her sister gave her a hand.

The ladies were astounded by what they found. 'It's not a cat, Alice. It's a . . .' She had it almost immediately. 'It's an armadillo!'

'It must have escaped from Regent's Park. Come on, get it into the house and I'll ring London Zoo.'

Still fuming over what young people were coming to, they carried the still living and, although they did not know it, severely shocked armadillo into their house in Arundel Gardens. While Alice went to the phone, her sister put the strange animal in front of the gas fire and wondered how to get something reviving into it. Its tiny snout was tucked hard into its belly. Perhaps if she smeared a little rum and butter on its nose . . .

In fact the armadillo hadn't escaped from Regent's Park, nor did Alice manage to contact anyone at the zoo at that late hour. So Alice telephoned the vet who looked after the two sisters' dozen well-nourished cats. He had qualified with Andrew Greenwood at Cambridge and, on learning that all the cats were in the pink but that a stray armadillo was in need of urgent attention, passed it over to me. After all, he reasoned, the two old ladies were staunch old-style Methodists and if they said it was an armadillo, an armadillo it was − even if it was by now pub turning-out time and an hour when vets in small-animal practice are accustomed to calls from revellers who return home with pink elephants to find the budgie wracked by some real or imaginary pestilence. I drove through the busy late-night London traffic and arrived on the stroke of midnight at the house in Arundel Gardens.

The old ladies poured out hot chocolate and the cats sat around in silence while I knelt on the hearth-rug and inspected the armadillo. Its scent glands filled the room with the characteristic bitter odour of armadillo. Shock had caused it to relax and unwind partially, and I could feel with my fingers the haematomas and the unpleasant crunching of the multiple fracture in the foreleg. While Alice held the armadillo I gave it an analgesic shot, a light sedative and some cortisone. It wriggled and scrabbled with its feet but only weakly, and when I started to swab its abrasions with an antiseptic it began to vomit.

'It doesn't look good at all,' I told the two women. 'If it's alive in the morning I'll give it an anaesthetic and see what can be done with the leg but I'm afraid . . .'

They produced a large wicker cat-basket for me to take the armadillo in. Alice had also rung the local police station to report their find, and just before I left, a constable phoned back to tell us of the likely origin of the injured animal. 'Look and see if it's got two small holes punched in the left ear,' he suggested. I looked and it had. 'In that case,' he said, 'it's been reported stolen by an animal dealer in Brighton.' He sighed. 'What will they think of nicking next?'

Whoever had purloined my newest patient may have been heading for Club Row or one of the other street markets where livestock, often of dubious origin, is offered for sale on a Sunday morning by flint-eyed, fast-talking individuals who claim to be 'breeders' – yes, even of snakes, parrots and, if necessary, armadillos – in order to evade the regulations governing the pet trade. Perhaps he'd got cold feet and disposed of his unusual loot behind the pub. Or could the mild-tempered little animal (a related species goes under the delightful name of the pink fairy) conceivably have made a run for it? Armadillos can scoot along on tiptoe quite rapidly and are accomplished swimmers. Whatever the explanation, and I don't know it to this day, the armadillo was in Notting Hill within twelve hours of being pinched.

If you think pinching an armadillo is unique, I can recall many more incidents where persons unknown made off with animal booty from zoos. Fish, small reptiles and mammals of the Pets Corner sort are sometimes taken by children or their parents. Fanatic amateur enthusiasts of exotica have been known to go to extraordinary lengths to steal bigger creatures, particularly birds and reptiles. Thieves who break in to grab livestock for its monetary value tend to concentrate on birds and will tackle anything from rare finches to eagles and bad-tempered macaws. Sometimes the object of the abduction is to obtain a ransom for an irreplaceable specimen: not long ago some villain successfully extracted a handsome 'reward' for 'finding' and arranging to return one of Marineland Majorca's talented roller-skating cockatoos. It must take some guts and know-how to snatch some of the beasts that disappear. Rattlesnakes, crocodiles and otters have been among some species kidnapped in recent years. Most surprising of all was the theft of two fur seals, a small but viciously-biting kind of sealion, from Scarborough. Perhaps if we checked the casualty departments of local hospitals after a theft, we'd find records of folk who had been treated for 'severe' dog-bites.

Back at home I put the still breathing but soporific armadillo into my office and turned the heating up. We would see what its chances were more clearly later that day. The armadillo didn't move from its basket during the Sunday but its condition didn't deteriorate further and I gave it some sustenance in the form of a glucose saline transfusion. The stocky little foreleg with its broken bone would best wait another twenty-four hours, I decided. By Monday the little creature had improved enough for me to give it an anaesthetic and manipulate the fracture. Since armadillos can hold their breath for as long as ten or twelve minutes, I chose a barbiturate injection rather than gas. When the patient was unconscious I explored the injured limb and, finding no easy way of pinning or plating the bone fragments with metal, decided to fix it with a cast of fibreglass. With Hanne extending the limb with all her might, I applied the chemicals over a web of plastic mesh in much the same way that one patches damaged bodywork on a car. Martin, Hanne's younger son, carefully splashed cold water onto the fibreglass as it heated up during the setting, in order to avoid burning the flesh beneath.

'Dilly', as we christened the armadillo, a female, was on her feet and exploring the corners of my office by Tuesday, the same day that the incident was mentioned in a small item in the local press. I tried her with some food of the sort found toothsome by most zoo armadillos – milk, hard-boiled egg and tinned dog-food. She slurped the stuff up from a saucer and drank as well small amounts of honey and water provided in the bowl borrowed from Lenin, our cat. Armadillos are generally great trenchermen, although in zoos I have found that their healthy appetites often lead to obesity.

The animal dealer from Brighton contacted me the next day and arranged to collect the stolen goods when she was fit enough to travel, but by the time he rang I was away up on the Lancashire holiday coast, following a call from Norman Rolands, the public relations consultant for Belle Vue, asking me whether I would be prepared to give a quotable opinion about a very strange species. For the next summer season Ripley's Believe-It-or-Not Company were opening an exhibition of incredible things such as 'fur-bearing fish', mermaids and other genuine as well as hoax beasts. Among the collection was a newly acquired stuffed specimen of North America's version of the Abominable Snowman, the Big Foot or Sasquatch. All I had to do was to examine it and say whether the Ripley 'corpse' was authentic or not. A small fee would be mine either way.

If, as I believe, the Abominable Snowman exists (I have more reservations about the Sasquatch), I would hate to think that one would ever end up in pickle or full of sawdust in a sideshow on Blackpool's Golden Mile, but Norman and I motored over to the exhibition and I confronted the seven-foot-tall humanoid covered with gingery hair. I was not impressed. Apart from grave doubts about the skin, hair, face and digits, I found no sign of sex organs! The Sasquatch was neither male nor female nor anything in between and, Nature having made no provision for urine to leave the body, the poor creature must have had one hell of a permanently full bladder.

The show manager was at a loss to explain the Sasquatch's asexuality although as we were leaving he mumbled something about the private parts have been shot off during capture! I gave the faked-up Sasquatch a regretful thumbs-down, collected my cheque and Norman and I drove home, stopping in Morecambe Bay to have a supper of exquisite potted shrimps in butter.

20

2

I adore dolphins and I'm all for good circus. Blend the two together, however, and you've got trouble. I first met the Swiss couple, Conny and Gerda Gasser, when they brought their travelling dolphin show to Belle Vue in the early 1970s. Former trapeze artists who had played the Palladium, they were now into marine mammals. Their professionalism in show presentation was undoubtedly the most polished in Europe and made the amateur stage-craft of most British marinelands look parochial by comparison. Gerda, a shapely blonde lady, looked stunning on stage and was developing into a first-class dolphin trainer while her son, Robby, had an empathy for sealions, particularly one big and ferocious South American bull called Adolf, which within a few years was to blossom into as unusual and spectacular a partnership as has ever been seen in circus sealion acts. Conny was the moving spirit behind the whole set-up, an entertainer through and through, one of an old Swiss circus family, the most generous, charming and good-natured individual in the European animal business and someone of whom I was to see a great deal, usually when there was big trouble, in the years ahead.

The Gassers and I became close friends through many a long hour spent wrestling with some ailing dolphin or another and then afterwards, when the work was done, relaxing together over a meal, for Conny and Gerda are bon vivants after my own heart, with a nose for the hostelry that has an outstanding kitchen. Together we struggled with dolphins all over Europe and as far afield as Singapore and Indonesia. Wherever the dolphin circus went, sometimes for a stand of only a day or two, I was likely to follow. Some seasons when the Gassers were touring France and

Germany, I flew out to catch up with them at almost every town they visited. Sables d'Olonne, Idar-Oberstein, Berlin, Walsburg, Mainz, Frankfurt, Mannheim, Hanover, Minden, Osnabruck, Bochum – on and on go the entries in my diary for just one season of touring when I was trying to keep up with Conny and his caravans.

Conny's Flipper Show was quite an elaborate affair. One wagon contained a sophisticated filtration system and automatic water-treatment room. Another was a deep-freeze and animal kitchen. A sealion pool was built into a third. There were toilets for the public, an office, a portable beer tent and a special truck custom-built to transport dolphins in water, as well as standard circus trailers for the staff, tenting, collapsible dolphin pool, emergency pool, seating and much more. Two dolphins and a trio of sealions were attended by a full-time touring complement of around twenty-five, including a teacher for any children accompanying the circus.

This may all sound very well, and so it is – except for the stars of the show, the dolphins. Moving these complex creatures from place to place frequently twice a week and over many miles produces a multitude of problems that threaten their well-being. Apart from the stress of the moves themselves, there are temperature problems, water, quality fish supply, quarantine and medical treatment difficulties. It never stops: power failures interrupting filtration and spoiling the refrigerated fish here, an inadequate supply of rusty-coloured water from the stand-pipe there, and the impossibility of doing shows in some town that has been covered with circus posters by the advance man, because the animals have got a touch of food-poisoning. The troupers' brave motto, 'The show must go on', is fine for humans but it imposes intolerable burdens on dolphins which anyway don't have much of a life, swimming in the limited confines of the portable pool and rarely seeing the daylight.

Conny did his best to look after his animals in every respect, but it was simply the travelling which took its toll, and with so many factors that he could not control short of stopping touring altogether, the incidence of illness was depressingly high. And, just as you might expect, when animals as specialised and complex as dolphins fall ill they don't go in for simple run-of-the-mill sort of complaints. How long ago seem the days in Rochdale when cows with milk fever were back on their feet two minutes after an injection of calcium, and dogs obliged by suffering from pneumonias that quickly responded to sulphonamides; by contrast, uncommon creatures seem to delight in winkling out uncommon afflictions to contract.

Where there are dolphins it goes without saying that there is lots of water, not just in the pools and pipework and water-treatment systems but all over the place: in the fish kitchen, splashed in the auditorium and on the trainers' platform and as vapour in the air. In this water various families of nasty bacteria like to dwell. Although killed by the chlorine used in the pool water, they can survive and breed remarkably rapidly in moist areas free of disinfectant. They aren't a major hazard to the health of man and other mammals, although occasionally one hears of a hospital ward or operating theatre having to be closed temporarily because one of these bacteria has begun to cause a spate of post-operative infections – the bugs have made their homes in flower vases on bedside tables or even in eye-droppers. They're particularly attracted to transplant patients whose normal resistance to bacterial infection has been removed by immuno-suppressive drugs.

To me and my dolphins this ubiquitous, water-sport-loving bunch of germs present a particular threat. First, they're capable of attacking a dolphin virulently and sometimes kill in a matter of hours. Second and most disconcertingly, they laugh at most antibiotics which can be tolerated by dolphins. Penicillin, streptomycin, tetracycline, chloramphenicol? The bacteria I'm talking about, a principal sort of which is named Pseudomonas, couldn't give a damn. Not only do the drugs not affect them, but by killing other germs in the host's body they may actually help the wily Pseudomonas to thrive and prosper.

Conny Gasser's little dolphin, Bubbles, had an encounter with Pseudomonas that I will never forget. And it all began with a love-bite. Folk may say what they like about rabbits and goats but in my book the most constantly amorous animal must be the dolphin. His famous friendliness may be unbounded but then so is his sexiness.

Dolphins start playing the mating game early in life and although they cannot actually breed until in their teens, they can be seen making passionate advances when only a few weeks old, not only to members of the opposite sex but with equal ardour towards their own sex and to creatures of other species. Poor old Cuddles, the killer whale at Flamingo Park in the early 1970s, was incessantly pestered by importuning dolphins one-tenth of his size who made the most intimate advances, sometimes in the middle of a show. As Cuddles elegantly rolled onto his back in the water and waved goodbye to his audience at the signal from his trainer, a dolphin displaying the most shameless passion would fling himself onto the whale's wallowing stomach and make his intentions painfully obvious. 'Ho-ho-ho,' the announcer would ad-lib in strained tones. 'There goes jolly little Flipper trying to get Cuddles to dance with him. Ho-ho-ho! Yes, I think Flipper's saying he wants to dance.' Dancing was the last thing on Flipper's mind. The small children were nearer the mark when they prodded the nearest grown-up and opined in voices of bell-like clarity, 'The dolphin wants to stick a carrot into Cuddles, I think, Mummy.'

Love-play among these lustful porpoises is often quite rough. They particularly fancy giving the object of their heart's desire light bites and nips with their teeth. Look at the skin of the dolphins next time you visit a marineland and you will see on at least some of the animals clusters of four or five parallel scratches. They can be found almost anywhere on the body and although almost always shallow, they do penetrate the skin. These marks of affection heal quickly and generally cause no trouble. Once in a while a tooth scratch becomes superficially infected and may need treatment from the visiting veterinarian.

Bubbles Gasser was undoubtedly a pretty dolphin to the human eye, but then who has ever seen an ugly dolphin? To her own kind, though, Bubbles must have had the uncommon appeal of a cetacean Bo Derek. Perhaps the curve of her dorsal fin or the tapering slimness of her tail-stock had about it that quality of line or evoked an eroticism in the macho dolphin bucks equivalent to, in human terms, Dietrich's legs or Dolly Parton's décolletage. Whatever the reason, she drove male dolphins wild with desire. Other females just didn't get a look in when Bubbles was in the pool, but apart from squabbling among themselves for her favours, her suitors were also a bit over-enthusiastic when biting the back of her neck or doing the dolphin equivalent of kissing her hand.

Dolphin flippers are not like fish fins; they are modified but otherwise typical land-mammal fore-limbs. X-ray them or dissect them and you will find the bones of the human shoulder, arm and hand. The finger bones of the 'hand' are very well developed and make up the major part of the skeleton of the flipper. The trouble began when Bubbles was lovingly but painfully bitten on her left hand, or rather flipper, by a rather pushy old roué called Fritz. Conny noticed that the four two-inch-long lines that were left as a token of Fritz's affection were becoming slightly inflamed. A day later the love bites had developed thin yellow centres and were showing all the signs of being infected.

When Conny telephoned me he described the yellow appearance of the tooth-marks – we had often seen it in the past – and I prescribed thrice-daily washing of the injured area with mercury soap and the application of nitrofurazone ointment to be protected by a thick smearing of sticky lanolin.

Three days more and Conny reported that Bubbles was eating and behaving normally but that the affected flipper seemed to be becoming puffy and the infected tooth-marks were expanding into broad, ragged, elongated ulcers. I keep reference books of the proprietary names used by pharmaceutical companies in the major European countries, so it didn't take me more than a couple of minutes to find the trade name for the antibiotic, lincomycin, used by doctors and chemists in Germany where Conny was then touring and to telephone through a prescription to a pharmacy in Bingen, the Rhineland town which was his next destination. Hanne was proving to be invaluable in such situations where sometimes my rudimentary German wasn't enough.

'Give the lincomycin capsules to Bubbles by slipping them into the gill-slits of a herring,' I told Conny. 'I'll fly out in three days time to see what effect it's had.'

'I'll be across the water at Rüdesheim by then,' Conny replied. Rüdesheim, the little wine town below the Niederwald where I used to go in my Rochdale days on the first weekend in October with Farmer Schofield, my next-door neighbour, to celebrate the Weinfest – it would be nice to go there again. It was 99% probable that the lincomycin working through the bloodstream would quickly have the localised infection under control, but I'd be able to make sure. Then Conny and I would be free to sample a trockenbeerenauslese or two.

As planned, I flew to Frankfurt, hired a Kadett and motored down through the roller-coaster countryside and the ever-somnolent villages that flank the banks of great Father Rhine. As soon as I arrived at Conny's blue and white painted encampment I went with him to look at Bubbles. His dolphin men brought her to the side and gently lifted her out in a canvas stretcher, then they placed her on a thick mat of plastic foam and I knelt down to examine the flipper. It didn't look at all good. The entire appendage was swollen and what had been the original tooth lacerations were now broad furrows of dead and suppurating tissue. Worse, the process seemed as though it might be deep enough to be involving the 'hand' bones. If that happened, and osteomyelitis became established, things could look very grim. Up to that time I'd had only one case of osteomyelitis of the dolphin flipper, in a dolphin belonging to my old friend, Reg Bloom, at Clacton-on-Sea. That had started in a deceptively innocuous way, had been recognised when we had x-rayed the limb and despite intensive care and medication had ended with Reg having one dead dolphin.

Cleaning the diseased area first, I numbed the skin with a freezer spray and then punched out a tiny piece of tissue with a special disposable sampling instrument. Part of this biopsy I would have cultured in the laboratory to see what bacteria were involved and the rest could be examined by a pathologist under the microscope. I also took blood for analysis back in England. Meanwhile immediate treatment was imperative. I had to assume that the flipper infection was caused by a tough organism resistant to the 'simpler' antibiotic drugs, and that one of the water-loving, awkward-squad of bacteria such as Pseudomonas was at work. Conny would have to haul Bubbles out of the water every eight hours for intramuscular injections of gentamycin, a drug that can destroy Pseudomonas and his ilk but which doesn't work if given by mouth. We'd found the chemical to be well tolerated by dolphins although, because of their massive kidneys, they needed three times the dose required by a human of the same weight. With gentamycin costing far more than many other antibiotics, a ten-day course would be costing Conny over £500 in drugs alone.

Conny isn't the sort of man to skimp on the medical care of his animals, though. Indeed, even when the animals could be purchased for a mere $300 apiece in the United States, I can remember only one example where a bad and unscrupulous owner neglected treatment of sick dolphins for reasons of expense and greed. That was in the West of England about eleven years ago, when we learned through the grapevine that an owner, well known to be in the dolphin business purely to make money out of the marineland boom raging at that time and without a scrap of concern for animals in his bones, was deliberately keeping quiet about two very ill animals in his possession. It was the end of the season. His plan was to let the animals die in the autumn, collect the insurance money and buy new animals next spring. No winter costs! As soon as we heard of this we travelled down to the dolphin pool, caught the animals and began their treatment with the help of a trainer borrowed from Morecambe marineland. Then we telephoned our contacts in the 'fur, fin and feather' group of underwriters at Lloyd's who specialise in livestock to put them in the picture, and sent a carefully worded letter to the miscreant making it abundantly clear that we knew what his game was. Happily, the two dolphins survived this attempt at murder by neglect, were eventually sold to responsible folk and are still alive and well in a famous zoo in West Germany.

We began the injections for Bubbles and I satisfied myself that Conny could administer the shots at eight-hour intervals as efficiently as a diabetic learns to cope with insulin syringes. In a week the circus would be in the city of Mannheim. I would come back and examine Bubbles there and then we would know the worst. Or, God willing, be out of the wood.

When I got back to England with my samples, Hanne told me that she had taken a phone call from a man who, she said, had an 'African' accent. He had enquired after Dilly, the armadillo whose broken leg we had put in a cast and who was soon to be restored to her owner in Brighton.

'He seemed most concerned,' said Hanne. 'Asked if the owner had been traced and whether the animal needed any special treatment.'

'Was he one of those kooky individuals who fancy an exotic pet, do you think?' I asked. Apart from a tiny proportion of people with a real interest and the ability to care for unusual species, the vast majority of folk who try to get hold of a monkey, big cat or bear to decorate the house, support their egos or impress the neighbours are either decidedly nutty or flamboyant showbiz types. Thankfully, the Dangerous Wild Animals Act now makes their efforts less likely to succeed.

'He didn't sound komisch,' Hanne replied. 'Rather nice and polite. Said he'd contact you later.'

Next day we were finishing lunch when the doorbell rang. I opened the door and found a tall black man standing outside. Behind him at the kerbside a long, black Mercedes limousine was drawn up with a chauffeur at the wheel and CD plates front and back.

'Good afternoon,' began the visitor. 'Doctor Taylor? I do apologise for calling without a prior appointment.'

'Please come in, Mister . . .?'

'I am X...... N......, from the Embassy in London of . . .' (he named a West African country). 'I spoke to your wife on the telephone yesterday. This afternoon I am on my way to Sandhurst where my son is at the military academy.'

My visitor was a heavily built man of perhaps fifty-five or sixty years with a face hewn into heavy features, broad ridges and deep clefts, with looming brows and a chin like a navvy's toe-cap, yet bearing a gentle smile. His voice was deep and vibrant, like kosher rum, Hanne said later, and his English was cultured though accented, as she had thought. He was well dressed in a dark grey three-piece suit and Homburg hat. A coloured fragment of ribbon glowed on one lapel and the big hand holding an ebony walking-stick bore a cherry-sized jade and red-gold signet ring. As he came into the hallway I saw that he walked with a pronounced limp and that the stick was no mere affectation. I took Mr N into the lounge and introduced him to Hanne.

'Will you take some coffee?' she asked.

'No, thank you, dear lady. I apologise again for this intrusion but I could not resist the opportunity.'

'Please do have a seat,' I said, speculating on the object of his visit. A new zoo in the capital of his country? A problem with some exotic pet that he wished to acquire as a present for a wife back home? Maybe even a query about the illegal trade in endangered species? It had happened before. I had forgotten for the moment that Hanne's caller of the previous day had talked only of the armadillo.

The African really was quite lame. As he lowered himself into an armchair he screwed his body round awkwardly to avoid taking any weight on his right foot and grimaced briefly. 'I must not take more than a few minutes of your time, but I am concerned about the poor armadillo that I understand you are caring for.' He took out a gold cigar-case. 'May I?' Withdrawing a long Imperiale, he guillotined the end with a gold cutter and struck a match. 'By chance I read in the newspaper about the finding of the animal,' he continued. 'What a strange place for an armadillo to turn up.' He smiled widely behind spirals of blue smoke. 'I had my secretary make some enquiries and here I am.'

'Are you interested in armadillos?' I asked. Aardvarks are the nearest thing to armadillos that are found in Africa. They are eaten in some parts of the continent, having been obtained, usually with great difficulty, by digging out their burrows, but otherwise I couldn't recall Africans showing much concern for these subterranean mammals.

Mr N's face became serious. 'Dr Taylor, I understand the armadillo was a, well, a stray.'

'Not exactly. It had been stolen. The owner has been traced by the police. An animal dealer in Brighton.'

'What about its injuries? Is it likely to recover?'

'I think so. It was severely kicked and has a bad fracture. But why do you ask?'

The African took out a cheque book and looked at me intently for a short while before answering. He seemed to be considering something. 'Because I wish to ensure that the armadillo has any treatment it needs. The best. No matter what. I will provide the funds.'

'But it will get everything it requires anyway. The dealer will receive an account from me.'

My visitor sucked deeply on the cigar and its fire glowed bright. Exhaling, he said, 'But are you sure? X-rays? Tests? Special drugs or equipment? I can provide whatever you need to ensure it recovers.'

An armadillo benefactor! The picture flashed through my mind of the armadillo tucked up in bed at the London Clinic with the Queen's Physician at one side of the bed and Professor Christian Barnard taking its pulse at the other while trolleys of specially prepared insectivorous food from the Connaught Hotel were wheeled in. I gathered my thoughts together and concentrated on the armadillo in question.

'At the moment,' I said, 'I feel that armadillo is doing fine – I'll show her to you soon – but I don't understand the reason for your generous offer.'

There was another, longer pause. Then, laying down his cigar, my visitor leaned forwards and began untying his right shoe. 'Doctor,' he said quietly, 'I request you to keep my name and indeed the circumstances of my visit in the strictest confidence.'

'Of course,' I replied.

He eased off his shoe and to my amazement began to roll down the silk sock underneath. When it came off I saw his foot – if you could still call the grisly mess a foot. Pink, white and black in parts, mis-shapen, with no sign of toes apart from a stump of the big one, it resembled an unformed lump of plasticine. Mr N cleared his throat. 'Do you know what that is, Doctor?'

Hanne had withdrawn. My mind raced. The grandmother clock ticked deafeningly. 'I...I think now I can guess. Old le...er...Hansen's disease, I think.'

The African nodded. He smiled gently again. 'You are right, Doctor, and you are also polite. Hansen's disease it is, to use its less emotive title.'

West Africa, South America – I saw the first glimmer of a link between them and the armadillo and this black man with one shoe on and the waiting Mercedes. The sound of the clock and the prattle of children outside as mothers took them across the fields to go shopping in Budgens echoed incongruously in my ears. Lightwater beyond the windows went about its business as I looked at the remains of a man's foot that had been ravaged long ago by one of the most feared and mysterious of all human diseases. Leprosy.

'I carry other reminders elsewhere,' said Mr N. 'All old damaged tissue. But I have had no active infection for thirty years, although I must keep taking the dapsone tablets on and off. Are you offended, Doctor? I do apologise if . . .'

'No, no. Not at all.'

'Only a few hundred years ago I would have been compelled to carry a handbell here in England and ring it constantly to announce my approach. Now I invade your home and stick my pathology under your nose. Am I not imprudent, to say the least?'

'I rather suspect that I should consider myself privileged that you have done so. I also think I see a possible connection between you and the armadillo. Ah! Here she comes!'

Hanne came into the room carrying the armadillo. Set down upon the carpet, Dilly proceeded to trundle around the room in a rather sleepy fashion. It was, after all, a time when respectable armadillos are curled up napping. The fibreglass cast was held out at an angle as she moved and caused her to hop along in a faintly comical fashion.

'So that is an armadillo.' The African watched keenly as Dilly made for cover behind a large ceramic leopard.

'You have never seen one before?'

'Never.'

He took a photograph out of an inside pocket and passed it to me. It showed a group of smiling Africans posed as if for an end-of-term snapshot. With them stood two white men in religious habits. All the Africans showed evidence of leprosy infection – thickened, distorted faces, gnarled appendages.

'White Fathers,' said Mr N, pulling his sock back on. 'At the leper colony where I found myself as a boy. I'm the one on the far right of the back row.'

I looked at the face in the photograph. It was almost but not quite unrecognisable, a caricature of the face of a punchy boxer just after he's lost a mean fight, but on a young man's body. I looked up again at the same face maybe forty years on. The chronically inflamed tissue had gone.

'Yes, it's me. Same fellow. I wasn't very pretty to look at in those days. God knows how many drugs I took over the years. First the awful chaulmoogra oil that gave me nausea, then after the second world war the sodium hydnocarpus treatment that really stopped my disease dead in its tracks, and finally the dapsone.'

Mr N explained that when as a youngster he had contracted leprosy, his family, animists by religion, had blamed the disease on their son's recent involvement with a nearby mission run by the White Fathers. The snake goddess had been angered by his leanings towards the Europeans' religion and his neglect of her rightful observances, they said, and had visited him with the dread sickness that would inevitably consume his body. The boy had been treated well at this mission, however, and cured in the sense that the disease had been halted, but there had been some irreversible bodily damage that the Catholic surgeons had not been able to erase; his terrible foot bore witness to the destructive power of the disease before the drugs had brought it under control. He had become a Christian and received a basic education at the mission. Through luck, hard work and guts he had done what few rehabilitated ex-lepers even partially achieve: he had returned to a normal life that soon made friends and colleagues forget what he had been. He went to university in France and, after qualifying as a lawyer, joined the government service back in Africa. When independence came to his country he rose with ease to a high position in diplomatic posts overseas. But he could not, would not ever forget.

'I have never in one sense left the mission at R......,' Mr N told me. 'Leprosy, Hansen's disease if you will, leaves scars, perhaps, if you're one of the luckiest, only small and invisible ones, but they are there, not only in the body but also in the spirit. I have seen many sad cases there which arrived too late for treatment – cases that the Fathers and doctors could do little for. I gave thanks to St Luke when I knew that the bacillus was driven from my body. I promised him many things – I know this may seem rather pi to you if you're not a Catholic – many things I have tried to fulfil. My debt is still immense. I owe a lot to the White Fathers who pulled me through as a young man and now, it seems, to the little fellow hiding over there in the corner. For now I read that scientists are turning armadillos into lepers to help in the fight for a vaccine against the disease. I see the need for vivisection experiments in medical research, but the idea of an animal being deliberately inoculated with leprosy germs – that fills me with the deepest feelings.'

His eyes glistened now as he spoke. I was totally transfixed by the unfolding of his story. I was listening to a man who had known suffering in a way that I never could. 'I must help in some way if I can,' he finished.

'But Dilly here isn't leprous and isn't going to be used for research as far as I know,' I assured him.

'I realise that, and I'm not trying to stop research. I just want to help, symbolically you might say, this race of new dumb lepers.'

'A gesture to St Luke or a propitiation to the snake goddess,' I said.

'Yes. Do you see?'

It was probably the strangest tale I'd ever been told by a client. It moved me and it did make a sort of sense.

There is still a lot of leprosy in the world. It occurs not only in Africa and Asia but also in Central and South America, northern Australia and, very rarely, Spain. Research is aimed at many aspects of the misunderstood disease that is universally regarded with exaggerated and largely unnecessary dread. A principal objective is the development of a leprosy vaccine, but for many years researchers were hampered by the very stubborn refusal of the responsible germ to grow in the laboratory either in nutrient media or in experimental animals. It just wasn't interested in multiplying outside the human body, and even in humans, the apparent immunity of many folk who are in contact with leprosy sufferers over long periods is not understood. There is a kind of 'rat leprosy' to be found in rodents but in many respects it is not the same disease as that in people.

Then, some years ago, it was discovered that the leprosy germ needed little persuasion to attack and breed in the tissues of armadillos. Possibly it has something to do with their body temperature which is very low for a mammal at 30°C (other related animal families such as sloths are similarly cool-blooded). So all of a sudden the unassuming armadillo, which likes nothing better than foraging for insects, termites, worms and birds' eggs in the cicada-clamorous, scented nights of the South American countryside, found itself in demand as a new laboratory animal – a convenient, easily handled, conscript leper. Very recently leprosy has been discovered in free-living armadillos and the animal has also been found to be susceptible to several other human diseases including typhus, relapsing fever and schistosomiasis. Poor old armadillo!

There was therefore a kinship between the suave black diplomat and little Dilly and her kind. I nevertheless found it remarkable that Mr N cared enough to want to help this unfortunate representative of one of the more primitive mammal families. I suspect that if the man himself hadn't shown me his foot and the photograph, if I hadn't sat and looked into his gentle eyes and heard him tell his story of goddesses and priests and suffering, I might well have put the fellow down as another, if more exotic, of the so-called 'humaniacs'. As it was I felt utterly humble.

'Mr N,' I said eventually, 'you can rest assured that we will do our best for the armadillo. If the fibreglass cast is a failure and the fracture doesn't heal, I'll arrange for one of the orthopaedic specialists at the Cambridge veterinary school to have a look at her. If there is anything to be done that the owner cannot afford, I'll let you know. How does that suit you?'

The African gave me a gleaming smile and tapped his walking-stick on the floor delightedly. 'And you'll let me know how it, she, comes along, Doctor?' He passed me his card.

'I will with pleasure, sir.'

My visitor stood up and we shook hands. 'If I can ever be of any assistance to you, Doctor . . .'

'Well, in your part of Africa there are some of the biggest frogs in the world, Goliath frogs. They can grow as big as a fox terrier. There were some at a German zoo until they were accidentally poisoned by the pest-control service recently. I'd very much like a contact for catching two or three of those.'

'Leave it to me.' Mr N said goodbye and went out to his waiting limousine.

Dilly settled down with us very well and the dealer from Brighton came to collect her when she was fit enough to go. Mr N would be pleased to hear that her ultimate destination would be the nocturnal house in one of Holland's top zoos. I arranged for the armadillo to be brought back to me in three weeks time for removal of the cast. By then her bruising and abrasions had disappeared and she was able to scurry across our lounge carpet as if the fibreglass mould didn't exist. Getting such casts off is always more difficult than putting them on, and this one took half an hour's work with a small saw and dental forceps to remove.

Underneath, the shattered limb had produced a firm callus of new bone at the site of the fracture. Set down again on the floor, Dilly made for the nook behind the television set, the healed foreleg going strong. No need for further surgical interference! Hanne and I were both sorry to see the little armadillo for the last time and when she had gone I dropped a line to Mr N telling him of her recovery and her future home in the Netherlands.

A couple of days later a Mercedes limousine pulled up once again at our door and the chauffeur delivered an envelope bearing a diplomatic seal in green wax. Inside was an invitation to a reception at a certain embassy in Kensington, a letter of introduction to a scientist doing fieldwork on Goliath frogs in Africa and a little religious medallion of St Luke, patron saint of physicians.

It was beginning to look alarmingly as though the case of Bubbles, the Gassers' dolphin, was not going to end so happily. I was receiving daily telephoned progress reports about her infected flipper from either Conny or Gerda, and it didn't take long for us to realise that we were in big trouble. Skin was starting to slough off the diseased limb, revealing bad-smelling dead flesh beneath. Bubbles was showing increasing evidence of pain and difficulty in moving the limb and was beginning to lose weight. My laboratory results came in and showed that, sure enough, the Pseudomonas germ was in the flipper. Tests further showed it to be a strain resistant to all antibiotics except polymyxin, a drug we couldn't use as it has to be dripped slowly into the patient intravenously, and gentamycin. Ominously, the laboratory added that gentamycin was relatively ineffective in the treatment of the germ.

'What do you think? Can the gentamycin hold it?' Conny asked when he called after arriving in Mannheim.

'I hope so, but I can't be sure. How does it look?'

'Seems to be spreading. Not much skin left on the flipper. Looks a real schweinerei!'

'Is she eating well and moving easily?'

'I'm not happy with her today. She's just refused some excellent mackerel and has only taken two kilos of herring. And she seems for the first time, how do you say, gleichgültig.'

I put down the phone and called to Hanne who was bottling fruit in the kitchen. 'What's gleichgültig, love?'

'Couldn't care less, without interest,' she replied.

So now Bubbles was listless. Was the infection spreading into the body? I picked up the phone again. 'Anything else, Conny?' I asked.

'Just one thing, my friend. Gerda has just come into the trailer to tell me that some more of the flipper has fallen off and she thinks she can see bone.'

'I'll be out on the next flight,' I said. 'There's only one thing for it now.'

'What's that? Can you think of another drug that might help?' Conny sounded weary, and I knew that he wouldn't be getting much sleep between the eight-hourly injections.

'No, there aren't any more drugs. We'll have to amputate the flipper.'

Conny didn't say anything for a moment or two. Then he said, 'A dolphin with one flipper? Would it be able to swim?'

I'd never seen a dolphin handicapped in such a fashion; with no dorsal fin or half a tail, yes, but what indeed would be the effect of removing a flipper? I'd never even heard of anyone amputating one before, and although we had seen many animals which had sustained severe shark bites and lived to tell the tale, not one had been injured on the flippers.

'It should be OK, Conny,' I replied. 'They don't paddle with their flippers. They use them as sort of attitude controls, to assist banking. We'll discuss it when I arrive.'

I put the receiver down. That was all very well, but would an animal with only one flipper be able to turn easily? Might it not tend to go in circles or have difficulty in diving or ascending? And how was I going to tackle the amputation? What sort of anaesthetic could I use on a dolphin in a circus in the middle of Germany? The problem of Bubbles' flipper occupied my mind totally as I set out down the M3 to catch the early evening Lufthansa 727 to Frankfurt.

In my bag was a comprehensive kit of orthopaedic instruments but no general anaesthetic. General anaesthesia in the cetaceans is extremely difficult, since the animals' anatomy and physiology provide an anaesthetist's nightmare. You can't use injectable anaesthetics and if you want to give gas, a mask applied to the blow-hole won't work; the animal simply holds its breath and won't inhale the knockout mixture. Try putting an anaesthetic tube down the mouth into the windpipe and you'll find no entrance into the larynx; to get into the windpipe you have to reach down the throat with your arm and literally dislocate the larynx from its socket in the roof of the throat. Even when you succeed in getting a tube into the animal, you must be aware that the dolphin brain is not responsive to low oxygen or high carbon dioxide levels in the blood, that breathing is at long intervals and of brief duration and that the lungs are accustomed to assimilating air under pressure when the dolphin dives. In other words, the sort of anaesthetic machine that will send a man, dog, horse or chimpanzee into the world of dreams won't be able to cope with marine mammals. What you need is a very special machine fitted out with a device that can both simulate the normal physiological conditions of dolphin breathing and at the same time introduce significant quantities of anaesthetic gas into the animal's system. One such machine, donated by the US Navy, is at our disposal in Cambridge, but I was going to have to tackle Bubbles in Mannheim without the help of that kind of technology.

With injectable barbiturates, narcotics and other liquid anaesthetics known to be extremely dangerous in cetaceans, I had decided to operate using the only remaining technique left to me – local. With the same sort of drug that dentists use to fill teeth painlessly, I intended to block the entire nerve supply of the dolphin's flipper. That was why I spent the 1½-hour flight mugging up what had been published in the scientific literature on the finer points of the anatomy of the area. I hoped the books had got it right; there wasn't much on the nerve anatomy of the shoulder joint and flipper of the Atlantic bottle-nosed dolphin, and what there was went back many years.

Perhaps when I arrive I'll find things to be much better than Conny's led me to believe, I thought. Maybe the flipper won't look half as bad as he describes. Maybe that wasn't bone that Gerda saw, just some gleaming white connective tissue. With a bit of luck, I may be able to avoid surgery and try some applications of polymyxin cream, for example. Things had turned out to be rosier than I'd feared many times before.

When I arrived at the dolphin show in Mannheim and had Bubbles fished out for inspection I saw at once that there would be no easy option, no conservative escape. Gangrene had set in. The flipper was almost entirely dead and the junction line between the rotting and living tissues was only a millimetre or two away from the 'armpit' where the limb joins the chest wall. The flipper must be removed at once. We had no choice if Bubbles was to have any chance at all.

Amputation of animals' limbs is not a common surgical procedure for the veterinary surgeon. It is obviously impractical in the larger farm animals and horses and it is widely regarded as 'cruel' among pet owners. In actual fact there is nothing cruel or unreasonable at all in saving the life of a four-legged creature by reducing its 'wheels' to three. Most cat and dog amputees in my experience get around just as nimbly as 'tripeds' as do their quadruped fellows. The operation is generally uncomplicated, fairly short and without post-operative pain or difficulties. We had been obliged to amputate the limbs of a wide variety of exotic animals over the years, birds being the biggest group. In 1960 the Belle Vue director, Ray Legge, and I had fitted out a one-legged flamingo with a wood and rubber artificial leg on which he got around most satisfactorily. In a Dutch zoo there is a one-legged gorilla and, most surprising of all, a kangaroo that springs just as jauntily on one limb as he did on two. I'm certain that the majority of zoo visitors don't notice anything odd about these animals. Still the fact remained that nobody could predict whether a marine mammal similarly handicapped would be able to shrug off its disability so lightly.

The circus was set up on some waste land close to the city centre. Not far away was the schlachthof, the municipal abattoir where I had sometimes autopsied dolphins in the laboratories of the chief veterinarian, Dr Helmut Fritz, who both shares my love of dolphins and is a connoisseur of the region's hocks. I wondered whether to ring Helmut and ask whether it would be possible to operate at his place, but it was by now growing dark, I didn't want to move Bubbles too far away from the pool and anyway the abattoir wasn't really set up for cetacean surgery. I decided on balance that the least undesirable alternative was not to take Bubbles anywhere but to operate right there by the side of the pool, and at once. I would operate on the ground with my sterile pack of instruments laid out on a plastic sheet soaked in povidone antiseptic. It would be surgery under conditions like those of the battlefield, working inside the tent beneath the tiered seating and in dim light, but I was concerned to reduce stress on the dolphin to the bare minimum. The quicker she was back in the water the better, and with the drugs I was carrying I should be able to keep her calm and ward off any post-operative infection from the un-hospital-like environment.

It had begun to rain heavily and rivulets of water were beginning to snake in under the tent walls. Pools formed in places and we squelched about. 'I want a tarpaulin washed down with chlorine and water to lay her on,' I told Conny, 'and three of your strongest men to hold her while I block the nerves.'

Conny and his men didn't take many minutes to arrange things, then I saw Gerda standing a little way off, looking distraught with worry. The strain of watching the mutilation of her beloved Bubbles was likely to bring on one of her migraine attacks. 'Go back to your trailer,' I told her. 'We don't need you.' She refused to go. 'Well, then, make us some good coffee, schätzi,' I said. 'We'll be through in twenty minutes.'

Bubbles lay peaceably on her side on the tarpaulin. I listened to her heart through my stethoscope – thirty-six beats a minute, strong and regular; typically, Bubbles wasn't showing any sign of alarm at being on dry land. She had been handled for transport and medical examinations so often over the years that she knew she had nothing to fear from the humans who always eventually re-launched her.

'Right. Two men to restrain the tail,' I ordered. 'One man and Conny holding her trunk. Firm holds but no leaning or kneeling on the flexible chest wall. Keep your noses and mouths as far away from her blow-hole as possible – I don't want her picking up chest troubles from us.' Once I had numbed the operation site, one man to sit with his arm round her head, talking to her in quiet reassuring tones, would be all the restraint needed.

When everyone was in position I gave Bubbles a small injection of librium into the vein in her tail-fluke and waited for three minutes while she became ever so slightly dreamy and relaxed. Then, after cleaning the skin with antiseptic, I inserted a long needle into her shoulder. When its point reached the place where I calculated the first big nerve supplying the flipper to lie, I connected a syringe full of xylocaine and injected. I repeated the procedure at other points to make certain that every nerve was totally knocked out. Finally I introduced a quantity of the anaesthetic along the line of my intended incision. Bubbles took my pricks without the slightest fuss. I told the men they could relax, but asked for someone to keep spraying water over the dolphin at intervals to prevent her skin from overheating. While waiting for the local anaesthetic to take maximum effect I studied the advancing gangrene closely. I saw that in order to cut through good tissue that would be suitable for suturing and would heal well I must take the flipper off close to the chest. I decided to cut straight through the stubby 'arm' bone rather than take it off at the shoulder joint, because I had found that the continued natural secretion of joint oil sometimes hindered healing in limbs amputated at otherwise very convenient joints.

When I took up my scalpel to start the operation I could not ignore a slight shiver down my spine as I thought again about what Bubbles might do when she went back into the water. Drown on the bottom? Quickly I put such corrosive ideas out of my mind and concentrated on the patch of sleek grey skin beneath me. It shone dully in the tent lights.

In order to speed up the operation and at the same time stop bleeding, I decided to cut the limb with surgical embryotomy wire once I had severed the skin with my scalpel. Bubbles never budged and no-one said a word as I slipped the loop of immensely tough cutting wire round the root of the flipper and began to saw rapidly. It took only ten seconds. With the loss of barely a dessertspoonful of blood the gangrenous flipper fell away. I hadn't taken all that much longer than the surgeons of Nelson's day, who prided themselves on their speed of amputations – one famous ship's doctor of the early nineteenth century could deal in under six seconds with the leg of a wounded man held down by two of his mates and with rum as the only anaesthetic.

I searched the operation site for any sign that the disease process might have sneaked beyond my chosen incision; there was none. Then I dredged antibiotic powder into the wound and began to close it with stitches of absorbable dexon.

Gerda was back again, staring out of the shadows beneath the wooden seating with a pale and haggard face.

'Don't worry,' I said. 'Nearly finished. Dolphin operation wounds heal remarkably fast in the salt water. I'm just going to spray the stitches with some plastic film.'

'How has it gone, do you think?' Conny sounded hoarse. His shirt was soaked with perspiration. He hadn't noticed that his trousers were wringing wet through squatting on the tarpaulin now awash with a blood-tinged mixture of water, disinfectant and dolphin urine. Neither had I until I looked down at my sodden clothing.

'Very well indeed,' I answered. 'Caught in the nick of time, I believe. Now let's try her in the water.'

Carefully Bubbles was slid into her stretcher and then carried up the steps to the rim of the pool.

'Hold her over the side and when I give the word roll her into the water,' I instructed the men. 'Tip her so that she hits the water on her good side.' I waited for what seemed like an hour but was in fact probably about twenty seconds for Bubbles to breathe one more time in the stretcher. The other dolphins bobbed expectantly, heads out of the water. 'Now!'

The men heaved and Bubbles leaned over and plopped into the pool. Down, down, down she spiralled. We all craned over the pool-side, trying to see through the shimmering reflections of the lights on the swirling surface. Was that her or was the grey wraith that constantly formed and re-formed in the depths one of her companions? Dolphins are big creatures but even in small pools they often seem to disappear, to break up into flickering shadows, once they go underwater.

Shortly a dolphin surfaced and took a soft, explosive breath. By the notched rear end of his dorsal I could tell it was Fritz, the Casanova who had been the cause of everything. Another dolphin came up and rolled easily onto its back to display a plump pink belly. It had two flippers so that wasn't Bubbles either. I felt that shiver of apprehension again. Then a kaleidoscope of grey shapes that seemed to ooze and writhe on the bottom directly below where I stood suddenly began to coalesce. They merged into a single form that grew steadily darker: a dolphin rising. It must be Bubbles. Her head broke the surface and she arched her back, taking a strong breath and flicking her tail. 'She's swimming!' Conny shouted.

Sure enough, Bubbles cruised across the water in a straight line. I watched, heart in mouth, to see what would happen when she reached the side of the pool. There was a slight wobble in the water as she prepared to turn, then we saw her make a few sculling movements of her one good flipper and roll effortlessly round as she changed course. Left or right turns seemed equally easy after those few initial wobbles. She dived just as easily as ever, and then made a power ascent that seemed to need just a little of the rather unusual oar-like movement of her flipper. When she went on to demonstrate a turn combined with a dive and then came up squeaking and mouth open to demand her first post-op fish, everyone spontaneously started to cheer. Bubbles was going to be OK.

'Well, what do you think now?' Conny asked me, hugging me with one arm and Gerda with the other.

'I think she'll be just fine,' I replied, 'but any more love-bites on the other flipper that go like that and I'm giving no guarantees.'

In fact Bubbles, the one-handed dolphin, did make a full and uneventful recovery. She was not to survive long, however, and the risky life of a touring dolphin circus was too much for her in the end: a few months later she caught hepatitis and died after a brief illness.

At least I am happy to know that there are no longer any travelling dolphin circuses active in Europe. Conny and Gerda have settled down and built a permanent dolphinarium in the delightful hamlet of Lipperswil near the Bodensee. Just as I anticipated, since then the health of their marine mammals – sealions, dolphins and a super little killer whale – has been excellent. Bad, I suppose you might say, for zoo vets, but very, very good for the likes of Bubbles.

3

If parrots were people they would be insufferable. The most intelligent of birds, they are also the most idiosyncratic, irascible and self-opinionated. One can like a parrot, but I doubt that one can love it. Parrots are born with a choleric eye, a jaundiced view, a strident voice, fixed opinions and the means to make those opinions felt in the shape of a beak that makes the same sort of impression on a human finger as secateurs might on a chipolata sausage. Parrots live a long, long time and bear grudges equally as long. The individual who can develop the knack of working with parrots and enjoying it is uncommon among animal folk; one who is actually tolerated (I hesitate to use the word 'liked') by Polly and her ilk is rare indeed and must, one would assume, have carbon-fibre appendages, perforated ear-drums and some distant ornithological blood in his lineage that the family don't like to talk about.

Just such a guy was the Englishman who presented the performing parrot show at Rio Leon, a Spanish safari park where I did a good deal of veterinary work. Four times a day he would set up his props on the stage in the open-air dolphinarium and his scurrilous crew of blue and gold macaws and sulphur-crested cockatoos would ride unicycles, play 'Find the lady', fire candy-bars from miniature cannons and abuse the spectators throughout. The star of the show was Arthur, a forty-year-old parrot who could do all the routines with ease and, spectacularly, would fall flat on his back and lie motionless for minutes at a time when the trainer pointed a toy pistol at him and said 'Bang!' Unlike most performing parrots, Arthur wasn't easily put off his stroke by small distractions. Many are the feathered thespians who utterly refuse to go on stage or seemingly forget their cues if something as simple as the patter of raindrops on the roof above them or an unfamiliar object lying on the ground near the stage distracts them. Arthur was too much of a pro trouper to be like that. Anyway, Arthur adored the peanuts that he was slipped by the trainer as the show went along. His vocabulary was extremely limited, but then he wasn't supposed to be a talking parrot. Someone over the years had taught him to enunciate loud and clear just one single word: the rather rude Spanish epithet 'Cojones!' This can be roughly translated as 'Bollocks!'

While he was actually on stage Arthur kept his trap firmly shut, unlike some of his colleagues who liked to squint at the audience and revile them with screeches while they worked. When the others were doing their thing, however, with Arthur sitting untethered and uncaged on his perch at the back of the stage, he would occasionally make a pertinent comment. Just as, perhaps, the trainer praised one of the cockatoos for a nifty display of roller-skating and asked for the approbation of the crowd, Arthur would get a word in. 'Cojones! Cojones!' came his shout. Nuns supervising their day-tripping convent-school groups in the audience would glare along the rows of chortling children.

When the parrot show was over it was the turn of the chimpanzees. Pongo, Pablo and Pepe, three adolescent chimpanzees, would hold a tea party. While the trio tucked in to buns and lemonade, ending up with a hilarious assault on the trainer with deftly-lobbed handfuls of trifle, the performing parrots sat on their perches and watched. Only at the end of the day were the birds returned to their cages in the parrot dormitory close by the dolphin pool. Pongo, Pablo and Pepe were amiable little chimps; I'd treated all three for measles and drained Pablo's knee joint when it became septic. You could not imagine three better-behaved or more composed great apes. They regarded their trainer as an elder brother, took their medicine from their doctor without fuss or fright and stoically ignored the parrots with which they shared the limelight four times a day.

The trouble began with Arthur and it was my fault. One day I was doing a routine inspection of all the stock with Rolf Rohwer,

Rio Leon's director, who asked me to look at a lump that had developed very recently on Arthur's back. I inspected a furious Arthur as he sat on his perch under a sun-shade, and gave him a stick to lacerate while I tried to snatch a quick feel of the offending swelling. Incensed beyond reason by my prodding finger and chagrined at his mistiming of a couple of lunges with his beak that were intended to amputate my thumb, Arthur decided to hop it. 'Cojones!' he bellowed, and flew off. He landed a few yards away – squarely on the crew-cut head of Pongo, the chimp.

Pongo was sitting sedately at the table, the tea party finished and the audience filing out, when he was sat upon. Instead of squealing and flailing wildly at his uninvited head-dress, Pongo hunched his shoulders, bared his teeth almost apologetically and looked round at us with an expression of total disbelief. The trainer moved to retrieve Arthur. Arthur contracted his claws slightly to take a better hold on Pongo's scalp, crouched and did the unmentionable – in a neat green and white pile plum in the centre of the chimpanzee's crown. 'Cojones!' crowed Arthur gleefully, as the trainer took him back to his perch.

There I continued my examination of the parrot's lump. It turned out to contain nothing but air, and when I'd drawn it all off with a syringe the lump collapsed to nothing. I'm still not sure what Arthur's lump was – perhaps a rupture of an internal air sac that had worked itself to the surface. Whatever it was, it never recurred and Arthur was none the worse for being 'punctured'.

There must, however, have been something about Pongo's head that had fascinated Arthur that afternoon, for from that day onwards he could not leave the poor chimp's cranium alone. In the middle of the tea party, often during each and every show, Arthur would yell 'Cojones!', spread his azure wings and swoop unerringly onto Pongo's top-knot. Once there he took secure hold, though never digging in enough to draw blood, and stared defiantly at his trainer. Pongo would squat miserably beneath him, all interest in buns and lemonade rudely interrupted. The visitors loved it, particularly when the trainer made his predictable move to restore order and Arthur just as predictably said the naughty word and squirted his disagreeable little pile dead on target. Not once was Pongo seen to strike back in anger; it seemed as if he was nursing his indignation. Before long there were occasions when the audience would chant 'Cojones! Cojones!' back at Arthur. He seemed to enjoy whipping up his fans and to a really good packed house yelling his catch-word he would respond with a double-dollop of green and white if he had time before the trainer collared him.

'Strange,' I remarked to Rolf. 'He never lands on either of the other two chimps.'

'It is,' he replied. 'But I'll have to put a stop to it soon. Arthur isn't doing any physical damage to Pongo, but I've a feeling the chimp's as mad as hell inside.' Rolf didn't realise how very right he was.

The first sealion to come to our new home in Lightwater, and probably the first of its kind to set flipper in the village, was Gemini, Terry Nutkins' little female Californian. Gemini had been born at Woburn and her mother from the outset had shown no interest in suckling the youngster. Terry, one of Gavin Maxwell's 'Ring of Bright Water' disciples in his youth and an experienced otter and marine mammal man, took on the terribly difficult task of bottle-rearing Gemini using the special sealion-milk substitute of blended herring, double cream, oil and water. Cows' milk is taboo for baby sealions and seals as they can't digest the milk sugar it contains and soon develop serious bowel troubles if given it. When she was four days old Gemini became colicky and showed signs of bad abdominal pain, so Terry brought her post-haste down to me by car. I passed a stomach tube into her and poured down medicine while Terry held her on his lap sitting on a chair in my back garden.

Gemini quickly recovered from the colic and settled down well on her artificial diet, growing fast over the months that followed. Moving house with Terry when he bought his lovely old inn on the Isle of Skye, she progressed to become a television star with a keen following of millions of 'Animal Magic' viewers.

I was appearing regularly on 'Animal Magic' myself, and some of my happiest moments were working with Johnny Morris on the programme. Johnny and his producers, first George Inger and later Mike Beynon, were easy, delightful people to work for. The popular science programme with which I'd been associated for Yorkshire TV had been frenetic in production, but the atmosphere at BBC Bristol was relaxed and informal and the animals always came first.

In one series of 'Animal Magic' I presented items on some of the small invertebrate creatures that I find fascinating. Leeches, the medicinal sort that are still occasionally used in British hospitals and after plastic surgery, are a misunderstood, rather clean-living species. Now extinct in most parts of the country because of the familiar story of the impact of modern man on the rural environment, these blood-sucking green and orange worms are as deserving of conservation orders as golden eagles and ospreys.

To illustrate for the programme the way in which leeches feed, I obtained half a dozen of the beasts that hadn't had a meal for a month (they cost £2 a piece from a biological supplier) and applied them to my fingers in front of the cameras with the help of the antique leech applicators and jars once carried by every physician. I persuaded the leeches to take a bite by first applying a drop of sugar and water to my skin as per the instructions in an eighteenth-century manual on leeching. When the three microscopic circular saws in the head of each creature went to work on me it was not without a slight pricking pain. While the worms rapidly sucked at my blood, elongating and dilating in the process, I started my spiel to the camera about the cunning way in which these worms keep the blood liquid by secreting anti-clotting saliva and use a tame colony of bacteria in their bellies to digest their vampires' feast.

Suddenly I felt something warm and wet expanding under the palm of my hand as it lay on the demonstration table and I looked straight ahead into the camera lens. Glancing down, I saw to my horror that I was streaming blood from a small Y-shaped wound where one gorged leech had dropped away. The kiddy-winkies watching the show at tea time in millions of homes round the country would be getting a close-up view of a creeping pool of gore in brilliant technicolour.

I was just about to try to mask the scarlet horror with my other hand when the studio first-aid man, who had been standing at the side of the set and seen what looked to him like a massive haemorrhage, leaped in front of the cameras and began slapping gauze and cotton-wool about. While he dramatically did his unscheduled and unrehearsed display of wound-dressing, I continued to ramble on about 'these interesting little fellows that extract just a teaspoonful of blood without you feeling hardly anything'. I completely ignored the big man in the uniform who was wrestling with my hand. When I saw the video playback later, it looked as if he was all set to do an emergency amputation of which I was blankly unaware.

As a result of the leeches item I received a telephone call the next day from a lady in Derbyshire who wanted me to 'leech' a bad bruise on her leg: a bruise is fundamentally clotted blood, so a suitable condition on which to use the little fellows. I politely declined her request but she persisted, saying that her son was a doctor, her GP had given his permission and I'd known what she meant if I would only consent to look at the bruise. I refused point-blank to treat the lady; it isn't illegal for a vet to treat a human – although the law does protect animals from human doctors – but I had no intention of starting a side-line of medieval medicine with folk queueing up to be bled, cupped, blistered or cut with two strong men and a brandy-soaked gag as an anaesthetic. I did agree to give her some of my leeches for her GP to apply if he wished. She travelled to my home the next day and was shown into my office. The leeches were ready in a tin with a perforated lid. The lady, well dressed and in her early fifties, had no sooner sat down than she hauled up her skirt to display the most hideous deep bruise of the shin I could imagine.

'Please, Doctor,' she said, starting to pull down her tights. 'That's been there since I tripped over the dustbin six weeks ago. I've gone through hell. Please stick on your leeches.'

'But I can't,' I replied. 'The thing certainly looks bad to me, even possibly infected. I don't want to risk it.' I had no idea what effect leeches might have on an infected area and anyway I couldn't see them being able to liquefy already clotted blood in an old injury like this one.

'Feel it, Doctor, feel it please!' I gingerly stretched down and prodded the thickened black and red tissue. It was iron-hard. 'There,' she said. 'Now will you stick them on?'

Although leeches carry only their special digestive bacteria and are otherwise totally free of bugs, I did not dare risk stray bacteria from the air or skin surface entering the puncture wounds. 'No, definitely no,' I repeated firmly, 'but you are welcome to all my collection of leeches. If your GP is prepared to take the responsibility, let him unleash the little chaps. Here.'

I thrust the tin towards her. With a look of deep disappointment she took it, hoisted her tights and prepared to leave. 'I really would have preferred you to do it, Dr Taylor,' she said sadly as she went through the door. 'You seemed to have such a way with the worms on the telly. They really seemed to like you. Are you sure I can't persuade you to change your mind?'

I never heard from the lady again and often wonder if she persuaded her doctor to leech her and what the outcome was.

Demonstrating wild animals and particularly small 'creepy-crawlies' on television was much more satisfying than working with domesticated species. As well as the leeches I tackled mosquitoes, bird-eating spiders, scorpions and giant African land snails. One outstanding item required me to cook, serve up and then actually eat some of the odder 'meat' foods that people relish in other parts of the world. There were witchity grubs from Australia, woodlice roasted in salt, a Zambian canapé, locusts deep-fried like chips and, from the USA, the prize recipes from the All-American Worm Cook-In. Mike, the producer, insisted that at least some of these goodies should be consumed live in front of the cameras. I love edible snails, particularly done the Spanish way in a hot peppery sauce, and shellfish of most orthodox sorts, so I know it was illogical that I couldn't face the fat witchity grubs with their plump white bellies bloated with what I am assured is a honey-like syrup. Nor was I of a mind to crunch up roasted, salted woodlice that looked the spitting image of simply dead woodlice of the sort found on any greenhouse floor.

I voted reluctantly for the earthworms, which Pru, the researcher, and I had made into a rather super-looking cake, and the locusts. I was once in Singapore when a swarm of locusts descended upon the city streets. Within seconds every door seemed to be flung open and Chinese folk dashed out, screeching in delight at their good fortune. They scurried around picking up the locusts, popping them greedily into their mouths and swallowing them with gusto. After half an hour there were no more locusts in down-town Singapore than you would expect to find in sunny Wigan.

When it came to the point in the programme where I could put it off no longer, I steeled myself and stuck a locust into my mouth, abdomen end first. It was no great shakes. The deep-frying seemed to have dissolved everything inside the carapace of the insect and it was like biting on a thin tube of roast celluloid. When it came to the earthworm cake I bit my chunk and chewed away happily, for only Pru and I knew that we had carefully constructed and baked the confection with one segment totally worm-free and marked out for my eyes alone by strategically placed bits of vermicelli. Johnny Morris was not in on the secret so I watched with fascination when he decided, live in front of the cameras, to sample a piece of the cake. When he pronounced it remarkably nice, I could only agree.

My work seems to attract the attention of the media, and I have done a good deal of radio as well as television broadcasting. Only once, though, have I been foolish enough to try my hand at doing a radio interview in a foreign language. A baby dolphin had been born at Holiday Park in southern Germany. I went down to examine mother and infant and found everything to be fine. While I was in the dolphinarium a German radio station telephoned to ask if I would give a live interview 'down the line'. Wolfgang Schneider, the director of the park and a good friend with a fine sense of humour, took the call and assured the interviewer that I could speak fluent German. It certainly wasn't so, and I protested loudly while Wolfgang continued to impress the fellow with my ability to answer his questions effortlessly. 'I can't, you know that, Wolfgang,' I shouted from the pool-side.

He put his hand over the receiver and shook his head sternly. 'You can, I insist you can.'

'But I . . .'

Wolfgang was speaking once again to the radio compère. 'So that's settled, Herr Vollmeyer. Dr Taylor will answer all your questions about the new baby. I'll hand you over to him now.' Wolfgang stuck out the receiver towards me and, muttering, I took it.

The interviewer spoke perfect English. 'Now, Herr Doktor,' he explained, 'we go on the air in five minutes. Just before then we will call you from the station. Please be standing by. We will be on the air for around three minutes.'

'But you'll keep it simple, please. My German isn't . . .'

'Of course, of course. No need to worry. I'll just ask you how the baby dolphin is, that sort of thing. No nasties. No tricky ones.'

Well, I thought as I put down the phone and waited for him to call back, maybe I could speak enough German. I worked well enough in the zoos with it. Hanne and I spoke it on odd occasions at home. I knew the basic medical vocabulary with the words for things like 'pregnancy', 'womb', 'suckling', 'umbilical cord' and 'afterbirth'. Perhaps it would all go as swimmingly as the interviews on matters zoological that I'd always enjoyed doing for English radio.

On time the telephone shrilled and I lifted up the receiver. I could hear music, the ubiquitous 'Flipper' signature tune, and then my interviewer went into his introduction. I followed it well enough, and listened to him explain that I was on the line from Holiday Park. Then began his first question.

'Guten morgen, Herr Doktor.'

'Guten morgen.' I was doing well so far, I thought.

In German the interviewer asked, 'And how are things going with the new baby and his mother at the dolphinarium?'

I fielded that one easy as pie. 'Oh, very well. Mummy is well and baby is well. Mummy has much milk.' Brilliant, Taylor, I thought.

Back to my friend at the other end of the line and his second question. 'Erwarten Sie, Doktor, irgendwelche Schwierigkeiten?'

'Er . . . I beg your pardon?' I hadn't the slightest notion of what he'd said.

'Erwarten Sie, Doktor, irgendwelche Schwierigkeiten?'

This was awful. Here I was, alone on the phone with perhaps hundreds of thousands of Hanne's kinfolk waiting for my reply, my message to the Fatherland, and I hadn't a clue. 'Mummy is well and baby is well,' I said at last.

Slightly fazed but quickly recovering himself, the fellow came up with his next question. 'Herr Doktor, warum ist in der Gefangenschaft das Züchten bei den Delphinen so selten?'

He'd done it again. I hadn't the faintest idea even of the drift of the question. I picked up the word for dolphin and something about captivity. I began to sweat. 'Mummy is well and baby is well,' I pronounced desperately. At least the Volk should be assured that things are just fine.

I silently cursed Wolfgang. If I ever get off this line alive I'll never speak a word of the language again, I thought. But here came my indefatigable inquisitor yet again. Gott in Himmel! Hadn't he twigged yet that he was talking to an idiot foreigner? Surely I would make some sense of this one. If only he'd keep it simple!

'Herr Doktor, die Nahrungsaufnahme?'

Donnerwetter! Did he consider a word like that simple? Nahrungsaufnahme? What the hell was that? Ah well, perhaps they'd take me for an unworldly professor. I began to intone my mantra. 'Mummy is well. Baby is well. Mummy has much milk.'

That did it. The interviewer got the message and began a speedy wind-up. 'Vielen dank, und auf wiederhören, Doktor Taylor.' There was a buzz and the line went dead.

'How did it go?' asked Wolfgang Schneider after I put the phone down.

'If you listen carefully,' I replied, 'you may hear Johann Wolfgang von Goethe turning in his grave.'

Never again did I make the same mistake. A few years later when I was at Marineland Côte d'Azur near Nice, doing a piece for

French television, the English director, Mike Riddell, translated my words of wisdom as I went along. I was standing in the water among the massive elephant seals wearing rubber thigh-boots and doing a medical check-up of the animals in front of the camera. The idea was that I should give my medical bag to one of the big bulls, who was trained to rear up like a monster caterpillar and clasp it between his front flippers, and then get in close to the beast to listen to his chest with my stethoscope.

In the event the elephant seal threw my bag away, embraced me with his great flippers and pulled me tightly to him. I was nearly suffocated, the ear-pieces of the stethoscope were ground painfully into my ear-holes and water began to pour into my thigh-boots. 'Oh, for Pete's sake! Somebody get him off me!' I spluttered.

Mike continued his translation for the benefit of l'entente cordiale and the cameras kept turning. 'Dearie me,' he enunciated in perfect French, 'this chest sounds a bit rough.'

'Cut the cameras. I'm pissed through!' I yelled.

'Isn't he a lovely old fellow. I enjoy doctoring elephant seals,' continued Mike in French. 'What fun we're having today.'

The bull tired of our close association and opened his flippers. Putting his stubby snout down, he butted me smartly in the midriff and sent me staggering backwards through the water. I had almost got my balance back when I came to the steep slope separating the shallow from the deep part of the pool. Arms flailing, stethoscope wrapping itself round my neck, I descended, still steadfastly facing the camera, into the depths. Wringing wet and with elephant seal excrement daubed over my hair, I surfaced, cursing and complaining bitterly.

'. . . and this sort of thing is really all in a day's work. It has taken me several years to perfect my examination technique.' Po-faced, Mike concluded his translation of 'my' blow-by-blow commentary.

'You really will have to improve your French, David,' he observed later when I'd showered and changed my clothes.

'Bloody foreigners,' I replied. 'You better open a bottle of Dom Perignon. I feel ''la grippe'' coming on.'

54

The fascination which wildlife seems to hold for all the media has given me some interesting and enjoyable work, but the use of animals in films, for example, still causes problems even though it is much more tightly controlled in Britain than it is in the USA. Both Andrew Greenwood and I often act as consultants for television companies making films and we have had difficult moments. Designers, directors, producers: all or any of them can and sometimes do ask unreasonable things of animal employees. Some of them imagine that to pay a facility fee of five or ten pounds to the person who provides a cat or duck for a play or documentary gives them the right to do anything they like with or to the animal. Over the years I've had to dissuade eager young telly-persons in charge of making popular science programmes on ITV from demonstrating how washing the grease out of a mallard's plumage with detergent would make it become waterlogged and sink, and from releasing a couple of hundred white mice into an unsuspecting hallful of seated ladies in order to illustrate, cinema verité, a piece about human panic. Peter Grayson, a former director at Belle Vue, once lost a contract with a television company because he would not allow a friendly spaniel that he had loaned for a play to be kicked realistically when the script required one of the characters to lose his temper.

I should emphasise that such stupidity is not common in British TV studios. A programme such as 'Animal Magic', for example, which uses large numbers of animals both domesticated and wild live in the studio, treats its non-human performers with the utmost kindness and consideration. The producer leaves the last word to the animals: if they don't want to co-operate or put on their prettiest face, no-one compels them or slips them a tranquilliser. If the unexpected happens, so be it; Johnny Morris, the programme's presenter, is an animal person through and through and can cope cheerfully with most things.

There has been considerable debate within the veterinary profession recently over what is or isn't permissible with regard to the use of animals in films. It has been claimed, for example, in defence of the successful 'All Creatures Great and Small' series on

BBC, that all animal characters seen anaesthetised in the programmes were ones which for some legitimate veterinary reason required anaestesia at the time of filming. Whether that is true or not, I personally feel that sedating or tranquillising an animal, and occasionally even giving some other form of treatment, can legitimately and humanely be done for the production of either documentary or fiction film material. When Yorkshire Television's 'Don't Ask Me' wanted to show live the birth of some piglets in the studio, Andrew arranged to bring in a docile sow who was due to farrow round about the date of the programme. Just in case nature took its course and pre-empted him, he had a couple more good-natured sows due to deliver a day or two later standing by on their farms outside Leeds. Half an hour before the programme went on the air, Andrew gave the sow an injection of one of the new prostaglandin preparations and lo, when the cameras started to roll, eight vigorous little piglets were delivered with not a scrap of harm to either them or their mother.

I myself was involved with the filming of scenes for 'The Omen' at Windsor Safari Park. Three groups of animals would be shown reacting violently to the presence of the satanic Damian. They were the giraffes, baboons and lions, although the lion scenes were subsequently cut from the finished film. The giraffe scene was easy. The little boy Damian approached the animals, which had been attracted to the correct point on the paddock fencing by succulent bunches of evergreen oak held just outside camera shot. When the signal was given for the animals suddenly to 'recognise' the devilish infant, I waved a large coloured handkerchief furiously over the top of the cameraman's head. The giraffes predictably wheeled on their heels and loped away.

The scene of lions attacking the car in which Damian was being driven by his mother, played by Lee Remick, was also simple to set up. Windsor had at that time a bunch of car-happy lions who might well have been feline readers of *Motor Sport* or *Autocar*. It didn't take much to get them to charge a car. Some individuals had developed the habit, not infrequently seen in safari parks, of playfully biting the tyres of a moving car, neatly puncturing them with their canine teeth and deftly ripping the whole circle of rubber from the wheel before the astounded driver could say 'gearbox'. Although some parks on the continent had ruthlessly culled all tyre-biters at the first sign of such a habit, the Smarts at Windsor had first tried aversion therapy. They aimed to administer a mild electric shock to attacking lions by rigging up an old wreck with extra batteries that were connected to the metal framework of the vehicle and leaving it in a tempting place on the road in the lion reserve. It hadn't worked: the lions with the Michelin urge had continued to run after cars, their heads darting in a precise curve at just the right moment to score a bullseye, and the Trojan horse had been studiously ignored. For 'The Omen', putting some lumps of meat on top of Miss Remick's car was doubly irresistible to the big cats unwittingly playing their parts as augurs of doom.

Baboons on the other hand, while enjoying automobiles just as much as lions do, are simply awful actors. Tyres they do not collect. Cars for them are free rides, chariots to play with, containers for bigger apes who might, foolishly, lower the windows and be relieved of their goodies, and bearers of bright, shiny bits of detachable material (screen-wipers, wing mirrors, radio aerials and the like) which can be taken away for trophies or brief games in the sunshine. Cars, in short, are good news, fun. Baboons adore cars and approach them amicably, so how to persuade them to attack viciously a saloon apparently carting around the devil incarnate? We solved this by heavily sedating a desirable young female baboon and carrying her, displayed plainly at the window behind Lee Remick's head, through the reserve. The reaction of the baboon colony was amazing. Thinking we were literally kidnapping one of their young ladies, they stormed the vehicle en masse and their rage was unfeigned. Howling, teeth bared, fingers clawing at the windows, they made exactly the spectacle the director desired. At rehearsal, however, two problems came up. One, Miss Remick could not drive the non-automatic car and her efforts quickly burnt out the clutch on the new Ford specially provided for the sequence. Two, Miss Remick refused to sit in a car that smelt profoundly of baboon excrement. The scene was eventually shot very successfully using Gary Smart, the young curator of the park, wearing Miss Remick's jacket and an ash-blonde wig with me crouched out of sight behind his seat holding the sleeping baboon up to the window.

When Twentieth-Century Fox decided to go to Iceland to film 'Quest for Fire', we were called in to look after what promised to be a whole range of animal problems. Elephants belonging to Jimmy Chipperfield and other circuses were to be transformed into mammoths by carrying ingenious costumes including false eyes, long tusks and shaggy coats. Lions were to be transmuted into their distant ancestors, sabre-toothed lions, through the nifty application of specially moulded sabre-tooth crowns to their upper canine teeth. I was prepared to anaesthetise the lions to take impressions of the teeth, a simple matter, but what worried me most was the art director's idea of making hard plastic crowns. Fixed with adhesive cement to the already long canine teeth, the extra length of the 'sabres' would produce enormous leverage and the danger of shattering the real tooth underneath. Jimmy Chipperfield and I insisted that the false teeth be fashioned from rubber, the producer agreed and we went ahead. Taking the impressions, using exactly the same materials and technique that a dentist uses for a set of NHS gnashers, and eventually fitting the realistic-looking 'sabres' turned out to be child's play. I didn't need to use a drop of tranquilliser or anaesthetic. The Chipperfields' big-cat trainer had such a rapport with his animals that he could hold each lion's mouth open long enough for the plastic mould to set perfectly round each tooth. Once equipped with their distant ancestors' impressive weapons, they seemed not to notice them and even dozed off peacefully. I cannot imagine many domestic cats putting up amicably with such dental theatricalities.

Hollywood doesn't treat animals in quite as cavalier a fashion as it once did. Cowboys' horses are no longer brought down, often with serious or even fatal results, by trip wires; instead, specially trained animals are used where such shots are required. Nevertheless, there is still much pitiless misuse of 'minor' creatures by directors in search of dramatic realism. Rattlesnakes, a valuable and much persecuted and misunderstood group of reptiles, have their heads blown off by pistol-fire in front of the camera and a hard time has been given in innumerable forgotten horror movies to vast numbers of bats and rats. The beheading of the water-buffalo in 'Apocalypse Now' was a disturbing example of prurient titillation masquerading as art and of murder in cold blood for the sake of the dress circle at the local Odeon.

Dr Marty Dinnes is the man who has looked after the animals' interests at many of the big Hollywood studios for a number of years and, apart from restraining directors and designers from indulging the wilder reaches of their imaginations where animals are concerned, he has made considerable contributions to the veterinary side of cinematography. From Marty I learned the secrets of dyeing wild and domesticated animals, how to give a blue rinse to a polar bear or to make a naturally chestnut nag into a glossy Black Beauty. Marty had found the way to colour an animal harmlessly for film work without producing skin irritation or damage and with a glossy, waterproof finish. It isn't as easy as you might imagine.

When a British film company wanted to use no less than two hundred black-as-midnight camels for an epic to be shot in Morocco, they were most disconcerted to discover that so-called 'black' camels are actually dark brown and hard to come by. Marty and I were asked to turn a great herd of ordinary camels into black ones. It can't be done by dipping them like sheep; the eyes and genitalia might be damaged by the chemicals and there are other technical problems concerning dyes in such large volumes. Marty instructed me in the only effective technique, which he had used on hundreds of wolves, horses and big cats. The process is similar to that used on ladies' hair and employs a colouring solution made by a famous American hairdressing firm, followed by hydrogen peroxide. A team of four men carefully applying the chemicals to a camel's coat can do about four animals per day and use around £100-worth of dyestuffs per camel!

Sensitive parts such as eyes, nostrils and genitalia are protected at the outset by Vaseline. I also learnt from Marty that the dye should not be applied to the skin of the scrotum. For that crucial area, and to ensure that it did not remain brazenly un-dyed and obvious on the otherwise glistening, jet-black body, clown make-up is applied – usually by the vet himself. Blacking-up a camel's private parts is at the best of times a hazardous operation and it is difficult to persuade one's assistants to reach between the hind-legs of a grumbling, regurgitating, side-swiping camel that has got its choleric eye firmly fixed on their every move. Some camel bulls need a shot of sedative before going to the coiffeur and we always use a full general anaesthetic when turning pumas into black panthers for jungle movies or grey wolves into the black ones that Count Dracula demands.

My work with the media has not always had a negative side to it. One particular 'Animal Magic' item concerning those jewel-like miniature helicopters, the humming-birds, showed me a fine display of what I might call practical birdmanship. The tiny luminescent humming-birds were brought to the studio by Len Hill, the celebrated founder of Birdland at Bourton-on-the-Water. After the programme had been successfully completed, it was time for the birds to be transferred from the studio aviary back to their transport boxes. During the transfer someone fumbled the handling of one of these record-breaking creatures (not only are they the smallest birds but they also perform the fastest wing-beats and produce more energy per unit of weight than any other warm-blooded animal). The little thing flew up and perched somewhere in the studio roof. We looked up into the intricate cat's cradle of gantries, runners, beams, lights, cables and walkways. Somewhere among that mass of steel was the minute bird weighing less than some moths at only one-twelfth of an ounce. There was no means of netting it up there.

'What on earth are we going to do?' asked an anxious floor manager. 'Won't it starve to death in here?'

Indeed it would. Apart from the effect of the low temperatures when the powerful lights were switched off, there would be no nectar or tiny insects, none of the food it required regularly and often to stay alive.

'I think it would be more humane,' I suggested to Len, 'to leave a man in the studio with an air-rifle to shoot it rather than let it starve up there.'

'Let me try a flower,' he said in his genial West Country accent. 'Get me a nice blossom or two.'

A researcher was sent off to find some flowers and returned presently with a rose and some freesias borrowed from the cafeteria. Len took a single freesia and held it up at arm's length towards the darkened roof. We watched and waited silently.

Suddenly there was a flash of bottle-green incandescence and Len covered the freesia with his free hand like a conjurer making a sleight-of-hand pass over an egg. When he opened his fingers at the door of the transport box, the minuscule humming-bird fluttered in a blur of wings back to its patient fellows waiting inside. The studio broke into spontaneous applause. Len grinned sheepishly and nudged me. 'Flower-power, eh?' he said.

4

If the chambers of Sir Arthur Conan Doyle's great detective had been situated in Hyde Road, Manchester, instead of Baker Street, London, he would have laid down his violin, lit a pipeful of rare Albanian Latakia and surveyed the evening fog rising round the speedway stadium beyond the window. 'I think, Watson,' he would have said presently, 'that this singular matter should be entitled The Case of the Italian's Peanut Butter.' 'A capital suggestion, Holmes!' the good doctor might have replied. 'For that, I recall, is how it all began.'

Each winter Belle Vue still puts on a famous Christmas circus. It used also to have occasional circus acts on site during the summer season. June had been unremittingly grey and rain-swept that year when, towards the end of the month, a team of footballing boxer dogs arrived from Italy to play for a month in a candy-striped mini-circus tent set up near the funfair. The owner, Signor Vamponi, arrived with one caravan for himself and his wife and one as quarters for the footballers.

The quarantine rules of Great Britain are strict and with good reason: rabies, arguably the most horrific disease known to man, hasn't been seen in these islands since 1902. The Vamponis had come from the continent, where the virus is steadily increasing its hold on the wildlife of many areas, so they had to quarantine their dogs like any other visitor, but the Ministry of Agriculture arranged for a building within the Belle Vue grounds, in which the two caravans would stand, to be designated as a quarantine area for the duration of the Vamponis' stay. It was inspected by Ministry vets and strict controls put into operation. No-one but the owners,

Ministry officials and the Belle Vue vet could enter the premises. The dogs could not be taken outside except to go straight into the nearby circus ring which was reached by a tunnel of canvas. All the dogs' exercising and bodily functions had to be performed within the designated quarantine premises.

I inspected the animals weekly on behalf of the Ministry, counting the dogs and checking each for signs of illness. After the first inspection, Signor Vamponi and his wife invited me to have a coffee and a glass of grappa in their untidy caravan. They were a picturesque couple, he small and swarthy with a Groucho Marx moustache and an addiction to snuff that had stained his nostril region brown, and she a tall blonde who had once been a Bluebell dancer until she had lost an eye in a bad car accident and had its place filled by a glass eye of electric blue; the impact of this unseeing, unmoving, gleaming sphere was increased by the fact that Signora Vamponi's good eye was brown as mahogany. Both spoke excellent English and regaled me with the latest gossip from the continental circus world: how an artiste had recently been strangled to death by a python he was working with in front of five hundred people (everyone thought he was hamming it up splendidly when he went blue and collapsed), how the glorious old Circus Bouglione building in Paris was still the same, and so on.

The Vamponi dogs were a cheerful bunch, keen players of the ball who were divided into two teams when in the ring, one wearing blue jerseys and the other red. The teams were kennelled at opposite ends of their caravan. 'Professional rivalry,' the Vamponis explained. 'They are highly competitive and have real team loyalty both on and off the field. If there is any squabbling among the dogs, it's always reds versus blues. Worse than Celtic and Rangers in Scotland, Doctor!'

As usual with circus acts at Belle Vue, food and certain other provisons for the animals were drawn from the zoo stores under the supervision of the redoubtable head keeper, Matt Kelly. Vamponi collected beef and some dog biscuits every day. Matt also came up with some fish, vegetables and a little fruit for the Vamponis' little pug who acted as referee in the circus act and suffered from mild diabetes that was controllable with careful diet.

One morning I was at the zoo to check on the progress of a young wallaby whose Achilles tendon I had repaired after an accident. The little marsupial wasn't recovering as strongly as I'd anticipated and I wondered whether some invalid food and peanut butter in the diet mightn't help to fortify it. I asked Matt for a jar of the peanut butter we kept in stock for such purposes. He shook his head.

'Bad cess to it,' he grumbled apologetically in his warm Dublin brogue. 'Wouldn't ye know ye'd ask for it today, Dr T. The Vamponis took both the pots Oi had this mornin'. We'll get more by this afternoon, though.'

I asked Matt if he thought the Vamponis were using the peanut butter to spread on their own breakfast toast. If so, they were definitely breaking the rules. The stores were for victualling the animals only. True, the boxes of bananas, pomegranates, melons and apricots, bundles of asparagus and broccoli, nets of onions and nuts, the trays of shrimp, sprats and herring on ice, all selected personally by Matt from the early-morning Shudehill market, wouldn't have looked out of place in the kitchens of the Midland Hotel. But a zoo must cater every day for a wider variety of tastes and palates than any chef de cuisine – carnivores, herbivores, insectivores and fruit-eaters, gourmands who will gobble anything and gourmets who are as fussy as an Egon Ronay inspector. The table d'hôte menu ranges from hundreds of bread loaves and gallons of molasses for the elephants to steak tartare followed by a fruit salad of apple, pear and chopped cherries for the iguanas. An entrée of cabbage heads and white mice must be prepared for the ostriches alongside snacks of hard-boiled eggs, locusts and nuts for the monkeys and more steak tartare, but this time flavoured with a few drops of formic acid, for anteaters who naturally insist on food which has the authentic aroma of ant. The danger is that such a cornucopia of goodies will tend to end up in human rather than animal stomachs if not carefully controlled. The keeper who munches the occasional grape taken from some dish he has prepared can soon progress to taking home a basket of greengrocery and a shoulder of lamb, and I've known places where an employee took enough each week to fill all his neighbours' larders. Apart from the financial loss to the zoo, the more dangerous effect is on the health of the creatures in his charge: malnutrition, even starvation, can develop while the office records still show a theoretically adequate amount of food being bought and fed to the animals. At Belle Vue it was up to Matt as head keeper to set up anti-filching counter-measures.

'The peanut butter moight be for that sugar-diabetic dog of theirs,' suggested Matt. It was possible. We agreed to overlook it this time.

A week later, still depressed by having lost my wallaby from a heart attack while I was removing the sutures in its leg, I was again at the zoo stores talking to Matt. The current problem was a weakly sitatunga calf that needed bottle-rearing. I had anaesthetised its mother in order to milk from her a few teaspoonfuls of the essential colostrum that the beautiful antelope calf had to have in the first day of life if it was to stand much chance against infant infections. Now I would give it to the baby by bottle and follow up first with protein solution and then with watered-down cows' milk.

'Let's use the normal human-type rubber teat,' I said to Matt, 'but with the squeezable plastic bottle. I think it will need encouraging to suck.'

Matt opened the door of the cupboard where we kept our special feeding equipment — premature baby bottles, stomach tubes, intravenous fluid sets and drenching flasks. We had the necessary tackle to pump bucketfuls of gruel into a convalescent elephant or provide artificial nectar to a humming-bird on the wing. He took down the box containing teats of various sizes, from baby mouse to baby hippo. Looking inside, I found that our stock of the size I needed was unexpectedly low.

'I thought we had more than these, Matt,' I said.

The head keeper muttered under his breath and screwed up his puckish face. 'Ah well, now. Vamponi borrowed some teats the other day for his dogs, after the shops were shut. He said he'd replace them. Oi'll see him about it.'

'The Vamponis again? Peanut butter and now teats? Have they been drawing anything else for their animals?'

'Well, just the usual meat and biscuits. Some milk. Oh, and some fruit and veg for the pug.'

'We can spare the odd apple, cabbage and what-have-you for the diabetic, that's legitimate. But I'm not having him nick our teats. Suppose we have an orphan cub tonight. Anyway, what does he need the teats for?'

Matt scratched his pate where it shone through the sparse covering of hair. 'Sure, Oi couldn't say. He said something about one of his dogs bein' still on the bottle. Oi was goin' to go and see 'em but you know the quarantine rules.'

'Rubbish! Those dogs are all full-grown. I'll mention it when I do my inspection tomorrow.'

Next day I was at the zoo early to take droppings samples from the sitatunga calf and then I headed for the dispensary inside the zoo stores to prepare a drench for the patient. Entering the stores, I almost collided with Signor Vamponi who was coming out carrying a large box full of bananas, apples, leeks and carrots.

'Oh, scusi,' he said, smiling, as I stood to one side to let him pass. He continued on his way without pausing.

'A fair bit of fruit there for your footballers!' I called after him. He said something that I didn't catch and kept walking. Ellie May, one of the elephants, deftly helped herself to a hand of bananas as he went by her paddock.

It was Matt's day off. In the store I found Len, the assistant head keeper. 'What's Vamponi doing with all that fruit?' I demanded. 'He had enough for a conclave of Vegans.'

'Claimed that they're for the animals, as per the contract with Belle Vue.'

'But a pug dog with diabetes doesn't need that much. I believe our Italian friends are scoffing the stuff themselves.'

'Maybe, Doctor. But what can I do? I'm not allowed to take the food into the quarantine area, nor is anyone else. If he says they need it, who am I to argue?'

When the sitatunga had been given its medicine I walked over to the buildings in which the two caravans were quarantined. I knocked on the Vamponis' door and the wife opened it.

'Prego, Dottore,' she said with a flashing smile. 'Come in, you are just in time for an espresso.'

Signor Vamponi was standing in the little kitchen area. He was working a coffee machine and gave me a cheerful 'Benvenuto'. The interior of the caravan was a scruffy chaos, reigned over by statuettes of saints and pictures of circus heroes. Clothes were piled everywhere. Unwashed crockery and glasses stood on tables and window sills. The floor was littered with bits of carrot and slivers of fruit peel and the pug scampered about in the debris.

'Please excuse the mess and take a seat while Alberto does what he can with this terrible chloriney Manchester water,' said Signora Vamponi, sweeping some filthy towels off a chair to make room. The air was stuffy and heavy with the odours of dog, coffee and butane gas.

'You'll find the boxers in perfect health, Dottore,' said Vamponi when we sat drinking his brew of aromatic Mocha.

'And you are keeping them indoors? No walks in the zoo grounds after dark?'

'No, no, Dottore, of course not. We understand.'

'How is the little pug with his diabetes?'

'Oh, still the same. Unless he steals a biscuit from one of the boxers or Laura here gives him a chocolate there is no sugar in his urine. But we carry the zinc insulin injections with us in case they are necessary again.'

'You can control him purely by a low carbohydrate diet?'

'More or less, Dottore.'

'Matt Kelly sees that you get fruit and vegetables for him, I understand.'

'Yes.' The Italian's face became abruptly unsmiling and mask-like. His wife stared out of the window and toyed nervously with the Ankh pendant hanging at her breast. They seemed suddenly tense.

'He seems to eat a lot,' I continued. 'Do the other dogs like fruit too?'

'Ah, si, si. You know, Dottore – a little vegetable and fruit each day is good for a dog. It gives plenty vitamins and, how you say, rough stuff for the intestines.'

True, and there are even cranks who believe in total vegetarian diets for dogs and cats. Such people find cats awkward converts to non-carnivorous diets but claim that they can be weaned into the right and proper path by titbits of cucumber, melon and fruit cake.

'So your footballers like bananas and leeks?' I went on.

'Love them, Dottore.'

'Cooked or raw?' I knew the stores were providing twenty cans of cooked meat per day and there was none of the typical smell of simmering stew in the caravan. Raw bananas might be acceptable to a dog but raw leeks?

'Yes,' said Vamponi. He was now plainly uncomfortable and began to tap a nervous tattoo on his knee with his coffee spoon.

'Raw?'

'Si, the bananas.'

'The leeks?'

'Yes . . . well, no . . . they are cooked.'

'You cook them and add them to the canned meat?'

'No . . . yes! Si, we cook them, don't we, Laura?' He addressed his wife petulantly in rapid Italian. She turned her head and looked at me icily, her eye of blue glass like the beam of a laser.

'Si, Dottore, cooked like Alberto says. Boiled, then mixed with meat, biscuits and fresh fruit. Is healthy, no?'

I changed my tack. 'Kelly says one of your dogs is still on the bottle but there isn't one under two years of age. Have you been over-generous with the grappa in his direction?'

Signora Vamponi gave a harsh, mirthless laugh from a mouth now trap-like and unsmiling. 'Madre di cielo, the man's mad. I borrowed a couple of rubber teats from him the other day for my friend, Rosa. She came to look round the zoo with me and brought her new baby. Rosa used to be with the high-wire Carvellos, but she married one of the Tower Circus clowns and lives in Blackpool now.'

I changed the subject. Slowly, warily the Italian couple relaxed again. So they'd been fiddling some food and some cheap teats from the stores. I could understand them being shifty. But their manner had puzzled me; I sensed it sprang from something more than such petty greed unmasked.

'Come, Dottore,' said Signor Vamponi eventually. 'Let us go to the dogs so you can write your report.'

The boxers were indeed in good health. No signs there of the weakness or tense hyper-sensitivity that can be the first indications of rabies virus newly arrived and rampaging in the brain cells. While I was going round the kennels in the dogs' caravan I sent Vamponi to bring me his copy of the import permit. As soon as he had gone, I pulled out of my pocket a banana and half an apple that I'd taken earlier from the stores. Quickly, before the owner could return, I broke the fruit into pieces which I pushed through the wire mesh to the boxers. Each dog sniffed the offerings and then utterly ignored them. Not one fragment was licked, let alone eaten. I couldn't imagine that they would have treated leeks any differently.

Back at the stores later I spoke to Len again. 'Stop providing fruit and greenstuffs for the Vamponis. They're free-loading on the zoo. If they want fruit for themselves they must buy it at the shops.'

No more greengrocery was drawn by the Vamponis in the days that followed but I was soon to hear of them again. I was driving towards the Dee estuary on my way to the Welsh Mountain Zoo at Colwyn Bay when a message came through over the radio-telephone. Would I please phone Boots the chemist's shop in Manchester concerning a prescription? I pulled up at the next telephone box to make the call.

The duty pharmacist came on the line. 'Dr Taylor? I've had an Italian couple in asking for an antibiotic – chloramphenicol suspension. No prescription. They said they were part of a circus at Belle Vue and have got trouble with one of their dogs. I explained that I'd need a scrip from a vet or in emergency a phone call. They got most upset when I wouldn't supply them with the stuff and said it was very important. So I rang the zoo and they put me on to you. Will you confirm the prescription?'

'No I won't,' I replied irritably. 'I know of no sick dog – anyway they're all in quarantine. Any sickness has to be notified to me and it hasn't been. I'll look into the matter.'

I thanked the pharmacist and went back to the car to continue the last few miles to the pretty hilltop zoo where a pair of Przewalski's horses awaited their regular hoof manicure under anaesthetic. After that I would call in at Belle Vue to see what the Vamponis wanted the chloramphenicol for.

Italy is one of those countries where anyone can buy anything, barring heroin perhaps, at the chemist's shop without prescription. I have a hypochondriac friend living in Rome who whenever he feels a cold coming on shoots himself up with an incredibly dangerous mixture of antibiotics including the controversial chloramphenicol, corticosteroids, vitamins, antihistamines and analgesics, all contained in one ready-filled syringe and purchased without a doctor's note from the local pharmacy. It's madness, of course. I could understand that the Vamponis might think that drug controls in the United Kingdom were similarly lax. Not so. There is enough over-use of powerful antibiotics with gay abandon by the medical and veterinary professions without laymen being encouraged to do the same.

'The Eyeties have been in again on the cadge,' said Matt when I got back to Belle Vue. He was bundling the week's harvest of fallen peacock feathers that had been gathered up from the park grounds by his keepers. The long plumes with their phosphorescent eyes would be sold to flower arrangers for £1 each.

'What have they been after this time – medicines?' I asked.

Matt looked up in surprise. 'How did ye guess? But so it was. Wanted some drugs for diarrhoea. Oi said they'd need to see ye first.'

I took some sample bottles from the dispensary and went over to the Vamponi encampment. The red team were running loose in the quarantine building while the blues, still locked away, barked disconsolately. Signor Vamponi, whistle in mouth, was giving the reds some coaching in leaping with all four feet off the ground for the shiny white ball. His wife sat on the steps of their caravan, fitting the pug out with some newly tailored black and white kit. Both greeted me with something less than effusiveness.

'Good day, Dottore. The medicine, have you brought it?' Alberto inhaled deeply over the back of a clenched fist and a small pyramid of brown powder vanished up his nose.

'I have come to see you about it, Signor. Why didn't you phone me if one of your dogs is ill? You are obliged to do so under the licence conditions, you know.' A boxer in hot pursuit of the ball cannoned off my legs and I found myself in the middle of the action with slavering, yelping players swirling all around me.

Vamponi lifted both hands level with his joke-shop moustache, palms turned outwards in supplication to heaven.

'But, Dottore, it isn't for the team. Is for Laura!' He swept one arm melodramatically towards his wife.

'Your wife? But you talked of a sick dog when you were at the pharmacy. Why?'

'Maledetto sia!' he cursed quietly. 'We thought we could buy some medicine for Laura, for her water trouble – how you say – cystitis? But when we asked the farmacista he says we gotta have a presc . . .'

'Prescription.'

'Prescription from a dottore. I say no but I know Dottore Taylor at Belle Vue. He will give me prescription for dog diarrhoea, no problem. Gotta keep the Italian dogs healthy, keep the British government happy, no?'

'So no dog is ill. No diarrhoea?'

'No'.

'But your wife has cystitis?' She looked perfectly fit to me, but that didn't mean she wasn't suffering from that common female complaint.

'Si, si. You understand?'

'Why not go to the medical doctor? It's free on the health service in England.'

Alberto frowned and I saw his wife look up, glower in my direction and shake her head. 'No is possible, Dottore. No time, so many shows today. Anyhow, she knows what she needs, what puts her right. Some liquid like the dottore in Italy gives her, chloramphenicol or terramycin. Laura can't swallow tablets.'

'Well, I'm sorry, Signor Vamponi, but I can't help. You'll have to see a doctor if you want that sort of treatment. I'm sure you could arrange for Dr Brown, the Belle Vue wrestling stadium MO to visit. Now, I'd like to inspect your dogs. Will you kindly blow the whistle for half-time and call the lads in.'

The Italians were beginning to annoy me with their hotch-potch of little lies and half-truths for the sake of a box or two of fruit, some rubber nipples and now some antibiotics. I had difficulty in distinguishing the true from the false in their Alice-in-Wonderland affairs. Penny-pinching, sly, dissembling – they acted more like gypsies than circus folk and to what end? I felt sure it wasn't mere stupidity. What I increasingly suspected was that there were more dogs in the Vamponi squad than I or the Ministry licence knew about. I counted all the red team and then went into the caravan to count the blues: twelve boxers in all. The pug referee made thirteen, all present and correct and apparently in tip-top shape, and with no sign of diarrhoea. But why would the Vamponis go to the trouble of not declaring extra dogs when they could have come in on the same licence? Unless they were ill – that seemed the likely answer and would explain the need for medicine and maybe for an invalid diet of peanut butter.

The building in which the two caravans stood was a mere shell of brickwork illuminated by a single window. No place to hide dogs there. If a contraband animal existed it must be in one of the caravans. The dogs' caravan where I was standing had been stripped of all its normal furniture and fittings; even the bathroom had gone. The interior was bare except for the kennels, one for each boxer, six painted blue at one end and six red at the other. The pug lived with the Vamponis, perhaps because a referee must always be seen to be impartial. The dogs' kennels were simple constructions of plywood and wire. I looked carefully at their dimensions as Vamponi brought one animal after another to me for inspection. False backs or bottoms in animal crates and boxes are commonly used by smugglers of livestock. I have seen six squirrel monkeys secreted

72

behind a consignment of as many macaws, and rare snakes in a hidden compartment beneath a chattering cageful of monkeys. A favourite ploy at one time was to smuggle valuable or prohibited small creatures concealed behind more lethal creatures such as cobras, big cats or crocodiles that the customs man and Min. of Ag. veterinary inspector wouldn't investigate too intimately. The only one of such smuggling incidents that I approve of was when a respected animal inspector now working at a safari park in West Germany brought his wife out of East Germany behind a group of very stroppy elephants who violently crashed the doors of their transport closed with their trunks whenever the communist border guards tried to look inside. You don't push your luck with opinionated elephants facing you head on!

Sadly, many of the animals illegally imported in such nefarious ways die in their cramped hidey-holes, not always because of lack of air or water or because of delays but from over-dosage of knockout drops given by the unscrupulous dealers in Bangkok, Kinshasa or Asuncion to keep them quiet when going through checkpoints. Could the Vamponis be playing at that dirty game? And for what – a litter of pups? Another footballer perhaps, some canine Pele, a star that they feared had a bad illness but couldn't bear to leave behind?

The kennels plainly couldn't have concealed anything much bigger than a flea. With one layer of plywood all round, each was built exactly the same. It must be the Vamponis' caravan then. The now taciturn and edgy Italian wasn't likely to invite me in for coffee and grappa this time.

'You go in ten days,' I said when we had finished the roll-call. 'It is necessary to begin preparing the export documents in good time. Is there somewhere I can sit down to do the writing?'

Vamponi scowled. 'Si, come into my trailer.'

I followed him into the other caravan and sat at a table in the lounge area while he searched for the necessary papers. There could have been space under the seating where a dog or two might be hidden away but there was no sign of any air-holes that might have afforded ventilation. Perhaps any ventilation was to the outside or under-surface of the caravan; I must try to look when leaving.

'I'll just pop into the bathroom if I may,' I said, and went over to the narrow door that was decorated with a ceramic plaque of le mannequin pis. A lavatory, shower, sink and tiny washing-machine were crowded into the minuscule room. I couldn't see how one could possibly attend to the call of nature, wash or clean clothes in such a press, let alone find space for a smuggled pooch. If, and I was beginning to have doubts, there were a sick dog or dogs in this caravan, they must be under the seating, either in the lounge or beyond, in the sleeping area. I flushed the toilet and went back into the lounge where I sat down heavily on the seating, making the framework shake. There was no hint of any scrabbling noise underneath me, but it was difficult to listen with a cassette player in the galley blaring Verdi.

While filling in the official forms I chided myself for playing amateur sleuth complete with *Boy's Own Paper* theories of skullduggery, dog-runners and secret compartments. The Vamponis were surely nothing more than a couple of strangers in a strange land. If there had been a little misunderstanding, the odd fib, that didn't make them mafiosi. They would be gone in a few more days, anyway.

Two days later I did indeed feel ashamed at ever doubting the Italians' explanation of their request for antibiotics. Matt informed me that Signora Vamponi had been taken ill and admitted to hospital for tests. Still, I reasoned, it wasn't my place to have given her chloramphenicol for her bladder trouble: leave that to Dr Brown. But the same evening, as I sat at the Keighley office going through the literature in an effort to find some information on the analysis of sitatunga milk (the baby wasn't putting on weight and I needed to change the formula of the bottle feed), I received another telephone call about the Vamponis. This time it was from the bacteriology department of Manchester Royal Infirmary.

'We've got one of the Italian circus people from Belle Vue in for observation,' said my caller, a bacteriologist. 'We've grown a culture from her and I thought you might be able to give us some information.' Cystitis isn't rare in dolphins and occasionally occurs in other zoo creatures, but the condition in female humans was outside my ambit, so I was doubtful. 'We've come up with a Salmonella bacterium,' he continued.

Salmonella isn't a germ particularly associated with the urinary system. 'That's surprising, isn't it?' I said. 'I know she has a history of cystitis.'

'Cystitis? She's not in here with cystitis. She was admitted with acute gastro-enteritis, suspected food-poisoning. We've grown Salmonella java from her sample.'

'How can I help you?'

'The source of the bug is concerning the public health boys. They're looking at some salami and mortadella that she'd eaten portions of and I've sent the original cultures to the central reference laboratory at Colindale for typing. You've had Salmonella in the zoo at times in the past, haven't you?'

'Yes. Last time in an elephant. Salmonella typhi-murium, probably from rodent droppings contaminating the hay. It died overnight before having a chance to show diarrhoea and despite a big shot of ampicillin.'

'You haven't any cases there at present?'

'None that I can find. The elephant was two years ago. I regularly screen each of the animal houses for background infection in the mouse population by hanging Tampax sanitary tampons in the drains for a week or two and then culturing them. No Salmonella found recently.'

'Could you take some swabs from the dogs they've got in quarantine? There might be a carrier there and we're keen to trace the source.'

'Sure. I'll do them first thing in the morning.'

When I telephoned the laboratory forty-eight hours later, I was told that all the samples I had taken from the dogs, and the salami and mortadella, had proved negative for Salmonella. 'No clues where the bugs originated,' said the bacteriologist. 'We must have missed something somewhere through I'm darned if I can think what it is. She hadn't eaten any shellfish, ice cream, meat paste or anything of that sort in the week before she became ill.'

'What did Colindale find?'

'No reply yet. Maybe tomorrow.'

Colindale's report when it did eventually arrive was a startling one. Signor Vamponi's Salmonella was no common or garden variety. It had been identified as type 01451227HB126, a variety so far unrecorded in Britain or Italy or anywhere else in Europe. 01451227HB126 was known to be resident at that time in the island of Borneo and to be causing a spate of intestinal infections in inland villages among the peasants. The physicians attending Signora Vamponi at Manchester Royal asked her about any possible connection with the Indonesian area. It turned out that she'd never heard of the place and had never in her life been farther east than the heel of Italy.

'Unless they're conning us again for some inexplicable reason,' I mused. The Vamponis were beginning to irk me once more.

Three days to the Vamponis' departure and it was time for the final health inspection of the footballers. Signora Vamponi was out of hospital, starting to work again with the act. 'I won't be sorry to see them go,' I said to Matt as we watched the sitatunga now drinking unaided from a bucket of artificial sitatunga milk.

'Oi agree. There's somethin' that isn't kosher there.' The Irishman lowered his voice. 'Personally, Dr T., Oi think they've been breakin' the quarantine rules. Havin' folk who shouldn't be there at all in the quarantine zone – maybe playin' with the dogs.'

'Why do you think that?'

'Your theory about smuggled dogs was off beam, Dr T., but suppose they've got an illegal immigrant tucked away!' Matt's expressive eyes were wide with anticipation. 'Charlie Entwisle, the security guard, reckons he's seen a kid in there. Looked through the window of the quarantine on his rounds last night and saw a youngster in the Eyeties' caravan!'

Entwisle was a tall ex-soldier with a shiny face of angry red crowned by a stubble of coarse yellow hair, and although his voice was loud and fearsome he couldn't run fast enough nowadays to back up the terrible imprecations that he hurled at the dozens of young boys who daily climbed the walls or ran through the gates behind delivery vans. He looked up as I tapped on the glass of his security hut by the main gate, and opened the window. 'Mornin' Doctor,' he said in his broad Oldham accent. 'Owt sick today?'

'No. What I wanted to ask you about was your seeing a child in the dog quarantine area. Is it true?'

The red face glowed brighter. 'Absolutely no doubt about it, Doctor. Saw the little beggar plain as a pikestaff in the Eye-talians' caravan skennin' through t'winder. Reet ugly little chap an' all. A proper little carrot-top 'e were, but pale-faced like a lot o' these sallow continentals. Unhealthy, Doctor. All that foreign food – spaghetti, macaroni, garlic an' that. Ugh!' Entwisle knew all about Abroad; he'd been there with the Eighth Army.

I was about to ask what time he'd seen the child when something flashed, bright as a magnesium flare, at the back of my brain. The lies, the things obtained from the stores, the medicine, the child, Signora Vamponi's illness – all the bits and pieces suddenly came together. Stunned at what I had deduced was the only possible explanation, I asked Entwisle to pass me the phone. Puzzled, the security man brought the telephone to the window and I dialled the Ministry headquarters in Preston.

That afternoon, when the Vamponis were in the middle of their football game before a crowded audience, I stood with a Ministry vet, a policeman and an officer of Her Majesty's Customs and Excise inside the quarantine building. The customs man was applying a gleaming stainless steel crowbar to the door of the Vamponis' caravan. With a metallic clang the door flew open and, led by the constable, we all entered. I was feeling troubled, to say the least, but my suspicions were stronger than ever. The Ministry man had shared them and had set up the dramatic break-in.

'The seating you think, Doctor?' said the customs man. He grabbed the nearest cushion and pulled it up. Underneath was a space filled with bedding. He moved along under the window and expertly dismantled the upholstery. More storage areas were revealed, filled with books, clothing, household items, fragile crockery packed to withstand travelling – all the impedimenta of travelling folk who needed to use every square inch economically, but nothing out of the ordinary. Dismayed, I watched as the search moved on to the sleeping area. Up came the seating, out spilled the blankets and pillows, night-dresses and pyjamas, even a pretty Victorian chamber-pot, but again no sign of stowaways.

The constable coughed a stage policeman's self-important cough. 'It seems apparent to me,' he said in his official voice, 'that we have been summoned here upon a misapprehension, a wild-goose chase.'

'Hold on, mate,' replied the customs man. 'I haven't even begun yet!' He went into the bathroom and pried with his crowbar at the base of the shower. It lifted and he got down onto his knees, bottom stuck through the doorway, and flashed a torch into the gap revealed. 'Nothing there but cockroaches,' he reported. Standing up, he looked around and then opened the refrigerator door. 'Wouldn't be the first time I've found one of these to be just a false front,' he murmured. But the refrigerator was a refrigerator and it contained only butter, eggs and some San Pellegrino water. Next he searched the cupboards but, apart from discovering where Signora Vamponi kept her jewellery in a secret drawer, unearthed nothing of note. A meticulous examination of the floor followed and likewise drew a blank.

The customs man was now looking as gloomy as the rest of us. He bent down, opened the door of the stove and flashed his light inside. No fire, just old ashes – but then it was supposed to be summer. Taking his crowbar again, he tapped the fire-brick at the back of the hearth. I heard him mutter something to himself and then he stood up, fished a retractable metal tape-measure out of his pocket and began taking measurements of the outside of the stove, the chimney-breast and pipe and the breadth of the caravan. He tapped several times on the stove-pipe and we heard its metallic resonance. Suddenly his calculations seemed to indicate something of significance for his expression brightened and he snatched up the crowbar yet again. He put the sharp bevelled tip into the joint between stove and chimney-breast and, grunting at the effort, swung on the bar. Slowly the stove moved away from the wall. We all pushed forward to look into the cavity his labours had exposed.

Three little orang-utans blinked back at us.

The Vamponis were heavily fined and the three orangs were confiscated by the authorities. All three were found a home in a good zoo where their Salmonella infection – the diarrhoea that the Vamponis had been hoping to cure with chloramphenicol and which Signora Vamponi had contracted in a more acute form through handling the animals – could be eradicated. Any home would have been better than the black recess behind the stove with only the stove-pipe as its venilator, where the little orangs had spent twenty-three hours a day for God knows how many weeks, only being let out in the evening and early morning to be surreptitiously fed milk from a bottle as well as fruit and vegetables and, when one became sick, peanut butter. If the Italians had bought the peanut butter, fruit and the teats at one of the shops just outside the zoo gates on Hyde Road they wouldn't have drawn our attention to them in the first place.

Smuggling great apes is a highly profitable business and it still goes on. Corrupt officials, many at the very height of the government, are everywhere in Indonesia. Everything from Komodo dragons to birds of paradise (exported as 'pheasants' with their tail feathers cut off and dyed black) can be obtained for the right price. Gorillas and chimps continue to come in considerable numbers out of African countries where only lip-service is paid to the principles of conservation, and their importation into European countries such as Belgium and Spain is virtually uncontrolled. Other European countries, Britain included, now strictly regulate what comes in and to whom it goes but there are still wealthy private collectors, some nutcases and a few disreputable zoo directors and circus proprietors who are only too pleased to pay several thousand pounds in cash, no questions asked, for a young great ape whose parents have been murdered to obtain it in Zaire, the Central African Republic or Sumatra.

Vamponi claimed that a buyer in England, whose name he never revealed, had welshed on the deal. If he wasn't lying and hadn't just brought the little animals to England on spec in the hope of finding a market, I'd dearly like to know who his mysterious client was. I'm inclined to think that on this point he told the truth.

Somewhere among us is a scoundrel, probably well-to-do, who deals in living creatures as if they were krugerrands or cocoa futures.

Perhaps, I reflected when it was all over, a more appropriate title for the case of the three ginger-haired orang-utans, if Sherlock Holmes had not already used it for one of his most celebrated investigations, would have been 'The Red-Headed League'. After all, as I said to Matt later, the Vamponi affair had largely been 'Alimentary, my dear Kelly.'

5

December of that year saw me back in Kenya, where a film was being made about Betty Leslie-Melville's work with Daisy, the Rothschild's giraffe which she had reared and re-introduced to the wild. Marty Dinnes rang from California to tell us that the baby giraffes gathered up for the making of the film, at that time using the working title of 'The Raising of Daisy Rothschild' but eventually released as 'The Last Giraffe', were in trouble. A couple had died, and others were ill. The American film director was in a panic. Shooting was being seriously delayed and stars like Simon Ward and Gordon Jackson kept waiting in the winter sunshine on the set outside Nairobi.

Now that I had been living in Lightwater for a little more than two years, I was beginning grudgingly to appreciate that the South, for all its lack of Pennine 'bite', mill-town friendliness and sense of distinct identity, provided some valuable advantages. One was that, although Manchester Airport had been an accessible jumping-off point for dashes abroad (and still is for Andrew), I was now within an easy twenty-minute drive of Heathrow and yet with thousands of acres of still, mushroom-crowded woods beginning just down the road. An hour after Marty's call I was boarding a Kenya Airways jet for the evening flight via Paris.

Before settling down in my seat in an attempt to sleep my way to Africa, I checked through my shoulder-bag. Always with me and packed with the basic essentials for an emergency visit of up to one week, the Bag can deal with the anaesthesia of around ten full-grown elephants and surgery up to the level of a Caesarian section. It provides containers for up to fifty samples of blood, pus or semen from mouse deer or from walruses. It holds enough pain-killer to ease a Bengal tiger with infected sinuses for at least enough time for alternative supplies to be located, and can begin courses of unusual antibiotics in critical cases where time is fast running out. It can also provide the necessary to stop me staying awake, falling asleep or getting malaria, prickly heat or a sore bottom. The Bag sees to it that, while I may not be up to Savile Row standards of sartorial elegance, I can keep warm, cool or dry, stop myself from smelling, and de-contaminate and wash myself after rooting about in the innards of a dying hippopotamus even where there is no water. In it I can find the wherewithal to purchase a falafel, fifty yards of net to catch a dolphin, a bed, an onward ticket to Acapulco or a five-peseta telephone call. It never runs out of credit cards, airline travel orders and ticket blanks. It even disgorges small but useful amounts of ready cash in the form of a tangle of dollars, dirhams, kroners, yen and even currency that normal self-respecting bags aren't legally supposed to come up with like Chinese ren min bi and Tunisian dinars. Yet with all this it is compact enough to travel as cabin baggage on an aircraft. Good old Bag!

Now, as the Kenya Airways plane lifted up into the darkness, I made sure that I had thrown into the Bag enough injectable valium, my preferred tranquilliser at the time for calming agitated young giraffes, and, because Marty had mentioned the possibility of abdominal problems, I calculated how many days supply of hyoscine I had and wondered what attitude the normally tough customs officers in Kenya would show if they opened the Bag. Then, as is my usual practice, I closed my eyes and mentally ran through a catalogue of common giraffe diseases, the treatments we had used in the past, the successes and failures, the drug doses on a body-weight related basis and the pitfalls awaiting the unwary who might use some forms of medication on giraffe that are normally totally safe and effective in other species. That completed, I popped a valium tablet myself, curled up and dozed off, thinking about earlier visits to Kenya and the little zebra, Tatu, whose cataracts I had operated upon there.* Was he still alive and able to see?

* See *Going Wild*.

The film set had been built up in the grounds of Jock and Betty Leslie-Melville's large English-style house in Langata. Now adult, Daisy Rothschild herself was too old to play the part of a giraffe calf and anyway she was roaming free with a small herd, although she regularly came back to the house of her human friends, often with one or two aloof boy friends in tow. The film people had captured half a dozen young Rothschilds of slightly differing heights, each of which would be called upon to play Daisy at a particular age. That was where the trouble had started. The giraffe calves were still only partly weaned. They had been moved to the film set with little if any acclimatisation to the world of homo sapiens, and not many days after arrival they were expected to tread the boards like fully paid-up Equity members.

Certainly no expense had been spared in some respects: Hubert Wells, one of Hollywood's most skilful animal trainers and handlers, was looking after the animals and he had a team of devoted girls working with him. The producer and the director and the cameramen, the actors and the technicians and the leggy girls who held clip-boards and cans of Seven-Up and didn't seem to do very much — everyone was most concerned about the band of baby giraffes. Concern, indeed, was in abundance. It was coming out of people's ears. It was keeping the telex machine in the Intercontinental Hotel hot with constant activity. It overflowed at the long tables laden with fruit and meat and fish that were set out under marquees for the film-makers by the location catering company. Concern, too, there was about the winter weather. Rain was about and the sun skulked for hours behind watery clouds. Back in the United States there was concern in the pocket-books of the men behind the movie, men who wouldn't know the difference between a giraffe and a jerbil. Yes, there was a cornucopia of concern, but not much understanding of what stress can do to young examples of some of the most delicate animals of Africa. The local veterinarian had been asked to knock the beasts back into shape when they had first shown signs of illness. Troubles had continued and the two deaths occurred. The concern in the film company, as the expense accounts rolled in and the baby giraffes faded away, took on overtones of panic. The Kenya government had specially licensed the taking of the Rothschilds for the film in the interests of promoting their conservationist image, but a Ministry official had made it clear that there were no replacement calves available if all the six expired. Concern in the hearts of the movie magnates on the West Coast had grown to coronary proportions. Dinnes had been contacted and now here I was.

After landing at Nairobi I drove straight down to Langata. The Leslie-Melville home is reached by leaving the main road and winding one's way down a track between plantations of banana and sugar cane and thickets of acacia, thorn bushes and the occasional baobab. The trees were dripping after a shower as I arrived. Climbing out of the taxi I saw to my great delight my first-ever wild hyrax, the immensely attractive, furry, cat-sized creature that is the elephant's closest living relative and the 'coney' mentioned in the bible. It was a tree hyrax, a common animal in many parts of Africa although rarely exhibited in zoos. It looked at me sleepily out of a hibiscus bush, its neck ringed with damp, glistening leaves, and made a remark composed of clicks and low grunts before pulling its head back and disappearing.

The house at Langata stands on land that rolls gently downhill to the trees and tall grass beyond the terraces and wide lawns. One could readily imagine when first seeing the building that the setting is Yorkshire or even perhaps the lowlands of Scotland; its grounds might most appropriately be surrounded by fells, dry-stone walls and fir trees. In fact it presides over a broad sweep of land that is pure Africa: broken bush with angular, sinewy trees, bushes with tousled hair, curly-crimped shrubs, yellow patches of grass that swirl with shadows, grey and agonised stumps, exploding gouts of dense green. And all of it alive and moving – mist shreds losing their grip at last on the tree tops, the heat haze vibrating like harp strings, far flocks of small birds rising suddenly from the savannah, dust kicked up by an invisible boot and settling just as quickly, black kites circling, wind and cloud and shadow gently playing tag, the distant landscape a patchwork of watercolours on a blanched background. Occasionally, a giraffe can be seen passing sedately between the trees in the distance and beneath them from time to time forages a lone warthog, one of Walter's family perhaps, or an industriously gleaning band of baboons.

I found the house and its immediate surroundings cluttered inside and out with the paraphernalia and personnel of film-making. It didn't take me long to find my contact, Clive, the associate producer. A charming though harassed-looking Englishman, he was obviously immensely relieved to see me, and as news spread that 'the giraffe vet' had arrived, I detected a change in the mood of the rather glum and sometimes tetchy members of the crew dotted around the house.

'Good to see ya, Doc,' the chief cameraman hailed me. 'When d'ya think we'll be OK for shooting with those babies?'

'What do you think's been up with 'em?' asked a man wearing headphones, a pink kaftan and a baseball hat.

'Say, Doc' — this from a girl invisible behind enormous one-way mirror sunglasses who turned out to be the film-set nurse — 'could you take a letter back for posting in London if you're going tomorrow?'

Everyone looked decidedly cheerier than when I'd walked in a few minutes earlier. I'd met the attitude often before among film and television folk: 'The giraffes are on the blink? So call the giraffe doctor. Get the guy in fast, pay him top rate and see that he replaces the dumb fuse or rewires the godamned circuit. No, it don't matter what it costs screwing a new gizmo into this giraffe, schmiraffe, so long as we get this show on the road by tomorrow! OK?' That is the general drift on such occasions. I suppose one might regard it as flattering, but I find it immensely irritating. Giraffes — or crocodiles or nightingales — are at least a million times more complex in their design and construction than the most sophisticated camera or television monitor.

'Don't you think I'd better have a look at the animals first?' I replied.

Everyone thought that a very sensible idea, and Clive took me over to the quarters that had been built for the young giraffes. Standing a little way from the back of the house, they were a cluster of small wooden pens each with a sheltered area. There was also a covered food kitchen. Four of the pens each contained a little Rothschild's giraffe. There is only one species of giraffe and its Latin name (Giraffa camelopardalis) reminds us that the mediaevals called the animal the 'camel-leopard', but there are within this single species many races and four principal ones. One of these, the Rothschild's giraffe, is to be found now only in quite small numbers, in north-western Kenya and south-eastern Uganda. The body-markings which distinguish the Rothschild from the other races are a tight network of white or pale yellow on a rich brown background of blotches over the trunk, and a more openly marked neck.

In the wild there is some interbreeding of giraffe races, but there was no doubt as I looked over the fence at these youngsters that they were all pure Rothschilds. Elegant, winsome creatures, with large blue-black eyes and outrageously long eye-lashes, they backed nervously away from me as I talked quietly to them. One of them, the biggest of the group and a male, seemed more apprehensive than the rest and adopted the strange star-gazing position I had often seen in uptight giraffes – head up in line with the neck which was bent slightly back over the body as the animal rocked agitatedly on its spindly legs. None of them looked normal and two looked positively unwell. The smallest female had severe diarrhoea, and both it and a slightly bigger female were completely off their food.

I asked Clive what sort of things he was hoping to film the giraffes doing. 'Dashing in a panic through barbed wire, being carried in an estate wagon, looking ill and limping among other things,' he replied and then added, inevitably, 'I suppose you'll be wanting to get back in a day or so. Have you got everything you need?'

I looked at the young female standing dejectedly as she passed yet another watery stream of faeces. There was an ominous flickering tremble of the muscles beneath the skin at many points on her body. 'Well,' I said at last, 'this one already looks ill, although you won't be able to film her like that. I'll need to get my hands on each of them, examine them and take blood. If you're lucky, we may avoid another death but it will be difficult.'

Clive looked aghast. 'But the filming! Can't you cure them, use something, give them a jab or whatever?'

'I need to talk first to the vet who post-mortemed the ones that died,' I replied. 'Then I need to see what the blood says. Meanwhile certainly we can begin treatment, but I must warn you that sick giraffes as young as this and so recently in from the wild are very tricky. I can't see me getting out of here, even if things go perfectly, for at least a week. And there's another thing – these animals won't be able to go onto the set for filming until I say so, and that means the next three days at the very least.'

Clive looked at the giraffe, now straining so hard that it had begun to prolapse an inch or two of rectal membrane, and slowly nodded. 'Whatever you say, Doc. Do what you need to do. I'd better find the director a triple shot of Chivas Regal and then go and break the bad news Stateside.'

He went off, and I was joined by Betty Leslie-Melville and Hubert Wells, the animal trainer. Both were very worried about the animals. Betty, who had done the original work on the real Daisy, has a special feeling for and rapport with giraffes. She contrasted the long months of struggles and setbacks that she and her husband had endured in fostering Daisy with the 'off-the-peg' system of intensive rearing that was being foisted for the purposes of the film on these gangling, wide-eyed stand-ins, and she didn't like it. She had had one or two dust-ups with the film-makers over the handling of the giraffes, and the relations between the two parties were obviously finely stretched. The deaths had been an especial tragedy for Betty for, although it was all happening on her property, the animals belonged to the film company and her contract did not allow any interference in the management of the young giraffes. Up to that point Betty and Hubert had been the only people with any significant knowledge of animals on the site, but it was plain that they didn't see eye to eye either on the subject of how to tend Rothschild infants. Hubert, whom I had not met before, was the man responsible for the care of the animals. Until I had arrived he had been receiving most of the flak over the hold-up in filming and, while glad to see me, he seemed at first a little suspicious of me and apprehensive, without justification as it turned out, that I might criticise his methods.

As so often happens, I found myself in a delicate political position. I could smell an argument in the offing so I diplomatically suggested that I should begin the examination of the only individuals who mattered – the giraffes – as soon as possible and slipped back to the house. I telephoned the vet who had done the giraffe post-mortem but gained little information of value: some congestion of the intestines, no signs of infection, nothing much else. Curiously, the vast majority of veterinarians in general practice in Africa know hardly anything about the diseases and treatment of indigenous wild species, and I find that the African students in the faculties of veterinary medicine at universities such as Nairobi have far less background knowledge of and interest in the native fauna than their European equivalents, although the academic standard is otherwise equally high. I decided to enlist the help of Dr Paul Sayer, a fellow Glasgow graduate and a first-class clinician working principally with the diseases of domestic animals in the clinical studies department of the veterinary school at Kabete. With a bit of luck, Paul could arrange for the processing of my blood samples from the giraffes. I rang him and he readily agreed.

Before examining the young giraffes I spent some time looking round the installation and watched the way in which the feeds were prepared. The animals had comfortable, draught-free and well-cleaned quarters and their diet consisted of powdered calves' milk substitute made up with boiled water and given by bottle, fresh-cut green foliage, hay and a little fruit. It all seemed reasonable, but I felt that the weaning process was being urged on too intensively; normally baby giraffes will suckle for ten months or more from their mothers, but the two sick ones here were only aged between three and six months. Also, although the giraffes' pens were supposed to be off-limits for all personnel other than those actually involved in their care, in practice there seemed to be a continual to-ing and fro-ing by the world and his wife for one apparently legitimate reason or another. Well-meaning folk coming to offer help, Africans carrying bales of straw and other supplies, VIPs paying a visit to the set: it might have been a quiet and sheltered corner of the Leslie-Melvilles' garden, but for the captive giraffes which not many days before had paced easily across the savannah beside their elders, drawn deep of their dams' rich milk in the pink dawn beside a papyrus swamp, and dozed in the murmurous midday beneath the acacias while the big bull kept silent watch, life was now strange and stressful. I talked to Hubert and arranged for the animals' privacy to be strengthened. Nobody, but nobody, except for the animal attendants and me was to go close to the giraffes. A lock was fixed on the gate leading to their pens.

The little giraffes weren't very difficult to check over. Hubert and one of his assistants patiently backed each animal into one of the corners of its pen which had been padded with straw bales. With one person on each side and a leather strap held across the animal's chest between them, they pinned it while I made my examination. I could feel the pulses racing and hear the hearts even without the aid of my stethoscope as the animals pushed against the restraining strap, nostrils flared and eyes wide. To take temperatures on fidgety animals that might well snap the ordinary glass clinical thermometer, I was now using an unbreakable electronic thermometer consisting of a thin, flexible, plastic-coated wire containing a heat-sensitive thermistor probe. The wire is inserted up the animal's rectum and the temperature registered on a dial. The whole thing is battery operated. I had had the wire for my thermometer made especially long, so that animals which like to jump about when strangers poke things up their privy places can do so to their heart's content while I stand well out of reach of hoof or claw. The longer wire also solved the problem of detecting fever in dolphins. Conventional thermometers can't reach far enough past the insulating layers of blubber around the dolphin's anus to contact tissues well-supplied with blood, so they always give a result that would seem to indicate the patient has frozen to death already. Now, using the wire probe device, I was able to reach well into the animal's body to record blood heat and had even for the first time taken the temperature of a killer whale with no difficulty.

After taking each giraffe's temperature with this instrument, prodding, poking and generally going over each animal, I took blood samples with a needle and vacuum tube from the large jugular vein in the neck and prepared swabs of the droppings for bacteriological examination. At this point I was inclining to the opinion that the essential problem was severe indigestion caused by the diet and general stress. Before releasing each animal I gave it an injection of hyoscine and another one containing the tissue-building and restoring type of anabolic hormone so beloved of Russian athletes. 'Cut out the fruit and water down the milk,' I told Hubert, 'and give the two worst ones, the ones with diarrhoea, no milk at all for twenty-four hours. Just warm water and honey and plenty of it.'

A driver took my samples to the lab where Paul Sayer had technicians standing by to process them as rapidly as possible. Typically it was by now early on a Friday evening, since all my urgent requirements for laboratory answers seem to come in the evenings at weekends. If I have blood from a cheetah that I suspect has been poisoned by barbiturate-contaminated meat or a biopsy from a critically ill porcupine with suspected liver disease, you can bet your bottom dollar it happens on a Friday night or a Saturday. If it occurs on a Monday, that particular Monday is always a Bank Holiday. On this occasion, Paul Sayer worked wonders and I was able to collect the results of his blood analysis the next day. Nothing much seemed to be out of the ordinary and there was no sign of infection or major organ failure. My patients were a little bit anaemic perhaps but that was all. The animals themselves seemed to be marginally improved although there was still diarrhoea, mopiness and lack of enthusiasm for food. Through the stethoscope I could hear unusually exaggerated activity in the intestines.

While I watched the first feed of the day being prepared the director appeared. 'How're we doing now, Doc?' he asked. 'Problem sorted out?'

'Not yet,' I replied.

He seemed a trifle sour. 'But I've got to begin shooting and every scene needs a giraffe. Doesn't your injection work?'

Any moment now, I thought, he will run true to standard form and start rattling on about some super-vet back in the USA who cures 100% of his cases in no-time flat with the aid of some purple pill and who would be pleased to help out if I cared to pick up the phone. I've found it to be an article of faith among laymen that in matters medical the second opinion is always the correct one and that the third opinion is infallible.

Sure enough the director continued, 'Look, Doc, if you think there's a difficulty here, I wonder if it might be a useful suggestion to . . . well, see, there's this veterinarian in Palos Verdes, Dr Farklewicz. Maybe you heard of him. We bowl together all the time. Treats Kirk Douglas's horses and did a fine job on Bob Redford's apaloosa stallion. He costs you an arm and a leg, but he's the best. See, I had this quarter horse on my ranch a couple years back. Exactly the same trouble as these critters! Now Doc Farklewicz gave some red tablets, can't remember the name, but barely an hour later that horse was . . .' The interrupting point arrived exactly on schedule.

'Yes, I'm sure that's so,' I said firmly, 'but this is a giraffe problem, and specifically a film company giraffe problem. The cause is no great mystery. I haven't been here twenty-four hours yet, but it's clear enough what's been happening.'

The director lost his sour look and raised his eyebrows hopefully.

'You've found the bug, Doc? One of these tropical viruses, eh?'

'No. Just human impatience pushing young delicate animals too fast. Somebody has the great idea to make a film, catch a bunch of baby giraffes to play the key role, no money is spared setting up the catching and holding operation.'

'Exactly, Doc. We've spent a bundle on this set-up, done everything for the animals' best interests. So how come . . .?'

'You did everything you thought necessary, I agree. But no-one considered the veterinary aspects of it all. These giraffes are under pressure. Artificial giraffe milk has been combined with a greatly speeded-up weaning process. Suddenly being dropped into close contact with man and kept in conditions of domestication – you can't imagine how much physiological stress that produces. No wonder the guts get screwed up. There's no virus or any other sort of exotic bug here – just stress. And the more you pressurise the animals the more risk you run of losing them all.'

The director took out a packet of Gauloises, lit a cigarette and inhaled deeply. 'So what do you think?' he said quietly after a long silence.

'Well, I'm going to ease up on the diet and change a few things. Give some more injections. We'll let the animals rest for a couple of days at least. Then we'll see. I'm afraid there's no alternative. It's my way or a film set complete with dead giraffes.'

The director nodded and gave a heavy sigh of resignation. 'Whatever you say, Doc. Maybe I can make it up to Lake Naivasha for a day sightseeing, then.'

When he'd gone I arranged with Hubert a gentler diet for the giraffes' still infant digestive tracts, with no fruit or vegetables, and injected each animal with a mixture of the metal called selenium, and vitamin E. By now, Andrew and I had seen scores of post-mortems of animals including wallabies, zebras, dolphins and birds, as well as giraffes, where the effects of drops in the levels of these two vital substances had produced fatal heart muscle damage. Finally I gave anti-anaemia shots. The little giraffes were perfect patients. As so often when coming to grips with animals either in or newly-arrived from the wild, I wondered what on earth they thought I was doing to them – sticking sharp points into them here, prodding there, feeling here. Of one thing I have long been utterly convinced: although the animal cannot have any conception of 'medicine', 'examination' or 'therapy', it so often seems to be able to differentiate between humans who harass, taunt or tease mindlessly and those who do things, sometimes unpleasant things, with good intentions. I can only assume that the beast senses consciously and, yes, possibly by ESP, the human attitude of mind.

When I am working abroad there is frequently plenty of spare time. I cannot and wouldn't want to treat the patients for hours on end unless there are special types of nursing, monitoring or trans-fusions necessary. Far from my home base I can't deal with any other cases except by telephone, so it is not uncommon for me to do only thirty minutes real work in a day. Although the telephone, telexes, making notes, official meetings and a limited amount of what might be termed public relations occupy several more hours, there is always time to enjoy being where I'm at. After the orang-utan has had its appendix removed and is sleeping off the anaesthetic or while I wait to see the first signs of response to injections give to a giant otter breathless and cyanotic with acute tuberculosis, there are the Velasquez and El Grecos in the Prado and callos, tripe cooked in spices, near the Puerta del Sol in Madrid, hot springs where one can simmer ecstatically in the frosty early-morning darkness of an Icelandic winter and the solemn, gold-glinting gloom of Nicosia's Orthodox cathedral.

Now, wondering whether Betty would have anything in store for me to compare with my meeting on my previous visit with Walter the warthog, I walked over to the Leslie-Melvilles' house. It was a warm, humid morning with a pale gold haze softening the landscape. Betty, slim and fair-haired, was standing on the terrace behind the house, holding a large blue beach ball. 'Would you like to see some giraffes play football?' she greeted me.

'Very much,' I replied.

Betty gave me the ball, put her hands to her mouth and began to call loudly towards the tree-line three hundred yards away. 'Dais-y, Dais-y. Come on, Dais-eeee,' she shouted. I stood watching the line where the lawns ended and the shrubbery of the bush began. Nothing stirred. 'Dai-seeee! Daisy Rothschild! Come on then. Cooooom on!' Betty was calling to the original Daisy Rothschild, now a free-living adult giraffe, just as if she were bringing the cows in for milking.

Suddenly I saw a giraffe head and neck appear out of the trees. Then another nearby, followed by yet another. Three stately Rothschild's giraffes moved quietly into view out of the undergrowth.

'That's a girl. Come on, Daisy! Cooooom on!' With great dignity the giraffes came over the grass towards us. 'The front one is Daisy,' said Betty. 'Then comes a bull, her devoted boy friend. The third is another female that we call Gladys.'

When they were about a hundred yards away the three towering beasts stopped and looked at us. Daisy may have been raised by human beings but the other two were one hundred per cent wild giraffe.

'They're not too sure of you,' Betty whispered. 'No matter, they'll soon get used to you. Here.' She gave me the beach ball. 'Take the ball and walk towards them slowly. When you're about ten yards away, give it to them.'

It sounded ridiculous. Approaching a trio of wild giraffe with a plastic ball! A giraffe weighs around a tonne and, because of its ability to 'pace' or gallop at great speed or strike lethally with heavy, sharp feet and horned head, has few natural enemies. So these three had nothing to fear from a puny unarmed homo sapiens but surely they would turn away from me with that typical giraffe aloofness. And suppose the bull was a little jealous of Daisy? I had been nearly brained by bulls that had suddenly flailed at me under similar circumstances elsewhere.

'Just throw it at their feet when you get near,' Betty instructed.

I walked towards the three immobile animals. They held their necks erect and looked down their noses at my approach, water vapour smoking faintly from their nostrils. Daisy, the nearest, was distinctly more relaxed than the other two. Her blue-grey tongue curled out of her mouth, licking her lips and preening her short whiskers. When I was close enough I stopped and threw the beach ball towards Daisy's legs. It rolled between her forelegs and she put her head down almost to the ground to look at it.

Then began a most remarkable display of soccer. Raising her head again, Daisy carefully tapped the ball with the front of a fore-hoof. It rolled a little way across the sward and stopped. Daisy walked lazily after it and played it forwards another few yards. Now it was the bull's turn. Was it my imagination or had he really seemed to relax as soon as I put the ball into play? He loped sedately ahead of Daisy, appeared to ignore the ball by staring into the far distance and at the same time kicked it sideways with a deft flick of his hoof. The ball rolled gently over the grass with the three giraffes in dignified pursuit. It was a most civilised game with never a hint of rough play, no particular sense of urgency and some apparent doubt in everyone's mind as to the direction in which any goal posts, if they existed, might lie. Daisy and her boy friend certainly monopolised the ball between them with Gladys rarely getting a look in, but her moment of glory came when she stopped a rolling ball by planting a fore-foot firmly upon it and keeping it there. There was no tackle; everyone stopped to look haughtily at the spectators and chew their cud. Then Gladys released the ball, the bull walked over and pushed it lazily away and the slow-motion game was under way once more. After half an hour of this the giraffes became bored and moved over to where Betty and I stood. The match was over and instead of lemon slices or pints of beer for the team it was time for rewards of apple which Betty brought out from the house.

It had been a unique and enchanting sight. Apparently the giraffes had started spontaneously taking an interest in football and no training of any sort had been involved. I thought what a sensation the leggy trio would have made coming out of the tunnel at Wembley on Cup Final day, but what tickled me pink was the fact that the African bush hereabouts apparently teemed with wild fauna that could be, as it were, sent for. I had been under the impression that only Tarzan could do that.

Next day the young giraffe patients were looking much better. They were all standing at the front of their pens, looking out with interest. Stools were returning to normal and I was particularly pleased to see the lick-marks on their coats where they had been grooming themselves with their long, abrasive tongues – a most important sign of improvement. Clive, the associate producer, was relieved to hear that we were unlikely to lose any more of the animals but I emphasised that I still insisted on at least two days without filming and even then I would reserve my position; when the giraffes were fit they could be used, but not a moment before. Meanwhile I gave them their injections at the 8 am 'sick parade' each day, checked their vital functions, inspected their coats for any signs of ticks and spent half an hour or so observing their behaviour.

When I had been on the film set for four days I decided that the giraffes were fit enough to do some brief, un-strenuous spells in front of the cameras. Clive and the rest of the crew were delighted to start rolling again and we discussed what pieces of action would be suitable for the first few days of the animals' return to stardom. We settled for a scene where a giraffe would put its head through an open bedroom window and nuzzle Simon Ward's hair as he lay in bed with his 'wife' and another where Daisy, represented by the smallest animal, would be carried in a minibus with its head and neck sticking out of the sun-roof.

The director was anxious to film another scene where Daisy had been lamed after charging through a low barbed-wire fence. What, he asked, was the best way to produce a 'lame' young giraffe without harming it? I said I would have to think about that.

Next morning we used the quietest of the baby giraffes for the bedroom scene. I had started to re-introduce fruit into the giraffe's menu in the form of over-ripe bananas, an easily digested source of valuable sugars. Hubey Wells and his assistants brought out the animal and patiently herded it over to the house for the filming. Everything worked perfectly. A sticky blob of brown banana pulp was hidden in Simon's hair, the giraffe was lured to the open window by Hubey with an armful of milk bottles and fruit, and with no trouble at all the scene was put securely 'in the can'.

The next take was to be the giraffe in the minibus. It had to be the smallest youngster as it was the only one that would fit into the vehicle, but I was rather worried about using that particular animal; it was without doubt the most nervy and highly strung of the group. I discussed the risks with Hubey. 'That's the one that might spook, right enough,' he agreed, 'and if it makes a dash for the bush, sure as hell we're not going to be able to stop it.'

I decided to use a valium injection on the little giraffe, just enough to make it calm without inducing grogginess. Calculating this type of injection is done very much by rule-of-thumb. Body-weight is important but there are enormous variations in the response by different species that can only be learnt by experience. Giraffes, for example, require about twenty times as much valium,

96

weight for weight, as do human beings. On the other hand, when using morphine, an elephant will be affected by a dose no larger than that normally given to a human adult. For sheer resistance to giant doses of conventional dope you can't beat the reptiles: I have known a half-pound turtle stay perky and very much aware of what was going on after receiving enough barbiturate in one dose to put an entire football team into a deep coma!

Setting up the gear for the taking of the minibus scene took most of the rest of the morning. While that was going on I found some potatoes and went down towards the forest edge and tried calling up Walter. He put his apoplectic-looking face out from behind the trunk of a whistling thorn bush after I'd almost hollered myself hoarse, but came no further. After sniffing the air he quickly dismissed all thought of me and my potatoes, pulled back and disappeared.

When the crew were nearly ready for shooting, I gave the little giraffe its valium injection and waited for twenty minutes. When the eyelids dropped ever so slightly I gave the word and Hubey gently moved it out of the pen. Again everything progressed smoothly. Under the tranquillising effect of the valium the animal walked unconcernedly over to the minibus and with hardly any coaxing was loaded exactly as the film script required. The tedious business of filming got under way and meanwhile I wandered around the site watching the design department assembling props for subsequent scenes.

A small triangular patch of ground had been dug up and its rich red-brown soil neatly raked. It was going to be the African servant's vegetable plot that is stomped over by a panicking giraffe in the film. To my horror I saw that the 'garden' was surrounded on all sides by gleaming rows of barbed wire. Of course! Clive and the director had said something about a giraffe running through barbed wire; that was why I'd got this sticky problem of faking up a lame animal. I shivered as I walked towards the wire-fenced triangle. This was ridiculous – barbed wire and the long smooth legs of a giraffe would make a grisly combination. Just putting the creature near the wire was asking for trouble and I'd seen and sutured too many typical barbed-wire lacerations over the years. What could the director be thinking of?

Only when I actually touched the wire did I discover how perfectly it had been counterfeited. It was film barbed wire made out of plastic and so cleverly constructed that it was indistinguishable visually from the real thing, even at point-blank range. I relaxed – but still I had the lameness to induce humanely. Smearing stage 'gore' on the giraffe's legs would be simple, but how to produce the injured hobble? Dogs and horses can be trained to limp and a pebble placed between the horseshoe and the hoof was the traditional method for producing fake lameness used by shady horse-copers, but by the time the minibus scene was drawing to a close I was coming to the conclusion that the giraffe's limp would have to be hinted at by clever cutting or simply talked about in the script instead of actually filmed.

As Hubert supervised the unloading of the utterly placid animal, I suddenly noticed how heavily it had been affected by the valium injection. The eyelids were now dropping almost to the point of closing, the tongue was beginning to loll out of the mouth and there was a slight wobble to its walk. Hubey urged it quietly to move back towards its pen. It rocked on its legs and began to hobble away, looking very much under the weather. My dose of valium for this particular individual had been a bit on the high side, it appeared. There was no danger, I knew, and by the following day the giraffe would have completely recovered from its chemical euphoria.

'Darling! That's abso-lutely divine!' The director's voice came braying at me from where he sat beside the camera, squinting at the giraffe through a monocular lens. 'Just what we need, Doctor. Freddy! Chas! Get those lights over there! Strike the set and move the whole bloody lot quick as you can, angels! Nigel! We've got our lame giraffe-kins! Fabulous! Doctor – can you keep him like that for half an hour while the sound boys sort out a gremlin?'

The little giraffe looked down somnolently as the crew hurried to set up new positions. It was quite plain from the look on the face of the director and the deferential tone of his minions when they addressed me that I was being given the credit for doing a neat fake-up job on the 'injured' animal. Not feeling inclined to disillusion them, I stuck my hands in my pockets, muttered loftily about it 'all being in a day's work' and thanked my lucky stars in silence.

When filming started again, a perfect sense of a lame and apparently shocked giraffe was captured with no trouble at all. As it shambled, ears down, across the grass I could almost see the torn tendons and shredded skin. The valium had neatly and precisely solved a knotty problem, but I made a note in my diary to revise my dosage rates for the drug when tranquillising young Rothschild's giraffes.

The animals steadily improved over the next few days. More blood samples confirmed their recovery and I decided I could go home. I travelled back to London with Gordon Jackson, a very lucky stroke: the check-in clerk at Nairobi airport was an ardent fan of 'Upstairs Downstairs' and, immediately recognising Gordon, insisted on 'Mr Hudson' and his friend being bumped up to First Class.

When we were back at home I telephoned Andrew to see what was going on; he had just got back from India where he had been looking at white tigers for Frans van den Brink, the Dutch animal dealer. After he had briefed me about his journey I asked him whether anything had been happening whilst I was in Kenya.

'Yes, bad news, I'm afraid,' he replied. 'Arthur fell into the dolphin pool at Rio Leon.'

'Arthur the parrot, the one who was giving Pongo the chimp such hell?'

'The very same.' Typically laconic Andrew. I always seem to ring my partner when he's sitting in his bath, and now I could hear over the phone the water splashing gently. (He is, incidentally, the only person as far as I know ever to have given a live radio interview by phone from the smallest room of the house.)

'That wouldn't do him much harm,' I said. 'He'd float and the dolphins wouldn't hurt him. Wasn't it just a question of fishing him out and drying him off?'

'No. He was in his cage when he went in. Trapped and drowned before they could bring him up.'

Poor old Arthur, I thought, gone down with his ship.

'Apparently the chimp, the one called Pongo, pushed the cage into the pool,' Andrew continued. 'Bold as brass, he sneaked into the parrot room after the last show when the trainer wasn't looking and stole Arthur in his cage. Taiji the dolphin made a vain rescue attempt and heaved out the cage, but too late.'

So Pongo, the persecuted chimp, had taken terrible revenge for past indignities, although Arthur had put up a spirited fight to the very end, it seemed, for Andrew was about to go out to Rio Leon to examine the nasty wounds on both of Pongo's hands that Arthur had inflicted during the tragic kidnapping.

6

Fire and ice, the extremes of temperature that can snuff out life. I've met both in my work with whales. The fire was the blazing sun of August in Malta where two young pilot whales had been found miraculously alive after no less than three days on the stone tables of Valetta's indoor fish market. They had lain there waiting to be purchased and killed in some way that doesn't bear thinking about, not for human eating but to provide mere fishing bait. A couple of hotel waiters had spotted the 'big black fish' early one morning when they went to the market to buy calamares. The two whales were puffing laboriously away in the cool air, their bodies hideously lacerated where they showed the effects of having been dragged from boat to market slab over stones and shingle and up several flights of steps. The waiters were no fools. Somehow they got hold of Windsor Safari Park's telephone number and called Gary Smart. Later the same day, Gary and I landed in Malta together with an assistant from the Windsor staff. For days we struggled to save the little animals, which must have been barely weaned when caught by the fishermen. The famous Phoenicia Hotel gave us the use of their children's swimming pool and there we nursed the whales, tube-feeding them with puréed fish, eggs and protein solution and anointing their wounds with healing cream.

Eventually we moved them to a bigger pool in the garden of an English couple living on St John's Bay. Things were going well by then; they were swimming more strongly, the blood analysis results were more like what I expected from pilot whales and the tube-feeding had given way to simple force-feeding of sardines and horse-mackerel. To protect the whales from sunburn as they cruised across the water or basked idly, we erected a contraption of wooden poles and sheeting over one end of the pool. A watch was kept throughout daylight hours with one of us ever ready to shoo the animals into the shade and keep them there with a net if they stayed too long with their backs out of water when the sun was high.

Eventually it became possible for us to relax. The whales were in such good condition that I felt we could begin to make arrangements to ship them to England, where we would prepare a good home for them at Windsor. Gary and I flew back to London for a few days, I to attend to other cases and Gary to set up the whale transport. While we were gone the whales would be watched over by Gary's assistant and by the two Maltese waiters who had by this time been bitten by the whale and dolphin bug, given up their jobs and set their hearts on a career in marine mammal husbandry. Before leaving I warned them about the need for vigilance against sunburn. The two little pilots were rather like British tourists newly arrived for a week's holiday on the Mediterranean, a bit too keen to get their money's worth of sun. They seemed to relish the warmth on their gleaming black backs and treated our shade with the disdain more usually associated with mad dogs and Englishmen.

When we returned to Malta I was horrified to find that our warnings about the sun had gone unheeded. The whales had been very badly burnt and the blisters on their backs were enormous. One blister alone contained a whole pint of clear fluid!

Gary and I were speechless with anger. When we at last found it possible to demand an explanation without committing mayhem, one of the Maltese told us, 'Yes, we did what you instructed, but the whales insisted on swimming back out of the shade into the light.'

'But then why didn't you keep them in the shaded part by using the net?'

'Ah, we had a better solution, Doctor.'

'What, pray?'

'Ambre Solaire.'

The English assistant that we'd left in Malta butted in. 'He's right, Doc. Here's the receipt.' He handed me a bit of paper. I read it: 'Vellas Drugstore. To supply 2 doz. botts suntan oil, £11.'

Ambre Solaire sun oil. For the whales. 'You used it on the animals?' I asked through gritted teeth.

'Yes indeed. Better than the net and the shade, we thought. Perhaps you're wrong, Doc. The blisters could be some sort of infection couldn't they?'

With a snort like an offended rhino, Gary stepped smartly up to the fellow and delivered the sweetest punch to his left ear. The chastised organ was, I swear, transformed into a red and succulent pepper within the second or so that it took its owner to collapse on the ground. 'Watch your lip, you bloody oaf,' snarled Gary. The two waiters backed off, wide-eyed.

'So you plastered the backs of the animals with the oil?' I continued.

Our assistant remained on the ground, nursing his ear. He nodded. 'Yessir. P-proper suntan oil, Doctor.'

There was no doubt what had happened. The specialised skin of the whales, its black colour particularly absorbent to radiation and the smooth swimming-pool affording none of the cooling spray and swell of the open ocean, had been literally fried in oil. The sun had induced what would turn out to be third-degree burns with all that that entails. The pain, shock and physiological disturbance caused by the pouring of blood fluids into the blisters predictably took their toll in the days that followed. Do what we might, from that point onwards the little whales were doomed. After another week first one and then the other died. We left Malta, the island where every second house seems to sport a dolphin-shaped door-knocker, in deep gloom.

Some months later came the ice. I was to find myself treating whales for problems caused at the lowest levels of the thermometer – no less than cold-loving killer whales affected by cold. No-one had ever imagined that such a thing could happen, and I was to break new ice in more senses than one!

It all started on February evening when the telephone rang while Hanne and I were playing one of our chaotic games of chess around a bottle of Pinot Grigio. Outside a loud-mouthed wind bullied the house with fistfuls of cold sleet. Andrew was away in Spain on one of the routine inspection runs through Majorca, Barcelona and Madrid. I looked at the clock as Hanne went to take the call. 8.15 pm. Hanne and I are pretty adept at forecasting who the caller is likely to be according to the time the phone rings. Although zoos and marinelands frequently employ night watchmen it is rare for trouble among the animals to be detected during the night. Consequently a bunch of my calls are related to the time when the keepers clock on early in the morning and go to their sections to discover a new-born antelope that is being ill-treated by its dam, a dolphin lying ominously still and upside down on the bottom of its pool or an eagle squatting stoically in a pool of blood, one broken wing trailing uselessly. So very early calls – 3 to 5 am – will be coming in from the Middle East, where they are four hours ahead of us and thus see their 'sick parade' not long after we go to bed. Around breakfast time comes any news of tragedy or disaster from British and European zoos, then we begin to take the calls which are usually from less urgent cases. Between 10 and 12 noon zoos have had time to distribute food to the stock and non-eaters will have been spotted. In the same batch we can expect the odd circus call – circuses work late at night and tend to sleep late in the mornings. Early afternoon is the most peaceful period. I have time to write and sort through my paperwork before the rush that starts at about 4 pm with the awakening of the Americans in the West; teatime is very much mid-USA time when I can expect consultations with friends in Michigan. Marty Dinnes and the Californians need a little longer to clear the breakfast things and come into action when there's an interesting item on BBC 'Nationwide'. The efficient Germans review the day's problems and like to discuss matters with me at length in mid-evening. Schneider of Hassloch, Tiebor of Munich's Florida Dolphin Show and Wurms of Stukenbrock are on the line then. Finally, as we go to bed it is the turn of the Far East and Australia. They are already into tomorrow and in the dawn glow over Jakarta or Surfer's Paradise have had a glimpse of something in trouble.

As Hanne reached to lift the receiver from its rest on the kitchen wall she placed a shrewd bet as to the identity of the 8.15 pm caller.

If she gets the person right I pay her 10p, if she only scores correctly on the country 5p. If she's wrong she owes me 10p. 'Jim Tiebor, München!' she called. She lost. It was a call from Iceland.

Saedyrasafnid is the small, rather sparsely stocked zoo and aquarium on the rocky coast a few miles from Reykjavik. It isn't particularly noteworthy although it generally exhibits a fine group of seals and has a couple of pools built to house newly caught killer whales. The director of the zoo, Jon Gunnarsson, was now on the phone and sounded to have a big problem: of five whales caught in the previous late autumn, one had died and the rest were ill. Could I please get up there as soon as possible?

When killer whales were first exhibited in marinelands in the late 1960s, Seattle in the United States was the centre for this capture. The groups, or 'pods', of killer whales which run each season between Vancouver Island and the mainland were encircled and corralled in those early days by catchers using half a mile of unwieldy and expensive stainless steel netting. By the mid-1970s techniques had altered dramatically. Not only had it been found possible to catch the whales on the high seas with trawlers deploying standard fishing nets, but Iceland had come to replace the North Pacific as the source for killer whales. Since then the Icelandic government has issued a licence for the capture of between four and eight animals each year to be undertaken by Jon Gunnarsson, an experienced ex-trawler skipper, and his team from Saedyrasafnid.

When Jon went off the line I phoned Icelandair and booked a flight for the following morning via Glasgow. Hanne helped me pack my bags and insisted that my first job on reaching Reykjavik should be to purchase a set of woollen 'long johns'. Although I hate the things I promised I would, but more important to me at that moment was worrying about what sort of equipment I should take for four ill whales. We cleared away the chess-board and I began overhauling my collection of custom-built giant hypodermic needles. Designed to penetrate thick blubber, they have shafts almost one foot long.

I arrived in Keflavik at the worst time of year for seeing Iceland. The lava fields crusted with ice formed a monotonous landscape under a leaden sky, wave upon wave of nature's industrial tips extending to an ill-defined horizon. The wind harried the treeless earth without ceasing. Stocky Icelandic ponies stood motionless as stones in fields of snow, broad buttocks taking the searing blast. Jon Gunnarsson met me at the airport and we drove at once through the wilderness to the zoo on the exposed seashore. Beyond the zoo towards Reykjavik lies the little harbour of Hafnarfjördhur, and the air reeked with the pungent smell of fish processing. A few terns wheeled above the roofs of the low wooden buildings that dot the hollows of the land, their paintwork weathered into soft pastel shades, the sea rolled black with its content of volcanic sand scoured from the shore, and a lone golfer in oilskins and a sou'wester leaned hard into the wind and drove his bright orange golf ball over the snow-covered links that adjoin the zoo.

Saedyrasafnid must be the most rugged zoo in the world. There you can see sheep and ponies that eat whole herrings mixed with their hay; Icelandic breeds long ago learned to survive on what little was available during the long winters. The polar bear pit presents a bizarre appearance in the colder months, when the pool water freezes solid. The bears, unable to bathe, become dark brown with grime, and the snow and ice of their quarters are red with blood from the dead seals provided as food. The bears are surrounded by countless objects that look at first like large brown butterflies. One quickly realises that these are the paired hind-flippers of seals, the only bit of the carcass which the bears do not consume.

Right at the sea's edge stand the high concrete whale pools. Jon took me over to look at the new killer whales. Jon's son, Gunnar, met us at the bottom of the steps leading up to the pool rim. 'Bad news,' he said as we shook hands. 'Another whale has just died.'

We climbed up to the viewing gallery. Up there the wind was even more vicious and cut through my parka as if it were made of silk. The pools were brimming with water that was whipped into a violent froth by the wind and sent stinging spray into our faces. Three young adult killer whales moved slowly through the water. A fourth was lashed to the wall to prevent its body from sinking.

'What did the first one die of?' I shouted against the gale.

106

Jon, a tough and genial character with a face and cut of beard that remind me of some Elizabethan soldier of fortune, took a generous pinch of the snuff that he uses to keep himself warm, and tapped his chest. 'Lung trouble. Pneumonia.' He pronounced the P. 'The vets at Keldur, the research institute, aren't familiar with whales. They specialise in sheep illnesses, but they feel sure it was P-neumonia.'

I would post-mortem the second dead whale as soon as possible, but first I asked, 'The other animals are ill also, you say. What have you noticed?'

'Slow, no interest, poor eating or not at all. And some sort of skin trouble.'

I squinted through the spray. Yes, as the whales surfaced to breathe I could see that the water didn't pour smoothly off their skins, which should have been like mirrors. Instead it ran away in cascades like water over a series of terraces. The skin wasn't smooth, and as my eyes became more accustomed to the spindrift, I could see patches of rough and jagged tissue on the animals' backs and dorsal fins.

'We'll have to drain the pool down so that I can get a close look at them,' I yelled, 'but first let's get the dead one out and to somewhere where I can do an autopsy.'

I thought about the 'long johns' Hanne had told me to buy; my legs were already numb with cold, but any shopping trip was postponed for the moment until after the examination of the dead whale.

I have to do many post-mortem examinations overseas and while some have to be done in far from ideal conditions, perhaps even without benefit of running water or shelter from the elements, I frequently have superb facilities put at my disposal by the local veterinary hospital. Iceland was a typical example. Dr Palsson, a distinguished expert in the field of sheep pathology and head of the country's veterinary services, readily agreed to me opening the whale at his institute. The sheer size of such a creature makes the dissection of a killer whale a laborious task. As they are too big to fit on a post-mortem table one has to break one's back working in a crouched-down position and then there is the problem of the disposal of the bits afterwards. Dr Palsson's staff helped with the sawing, provided warm water to thaw my hands when the cold threatened to make my fingers seize up, carted away pieces once I'd finished with them and brewed a steady supply of strong tea which they surreptitiously laced with tots of brennevin, the Icelandic answer to the Irishman's poteen.

What I found was alarming. Certainly the principal cause of death was severe pneumonia, but what was I to make of the skin? It was in a terrible state – dead, peeling and split to a depth of several inches over large areas. Looking into some of the wide cracks in the skin, I could see a glint of blood and blubber at the bottom. What had caused this damage? Not blows or cuts from solid objects during capture or when in the pool, nor rough handling in the nets, nor was this any kind of infectious skin disease, attack by bacteria or the ubiquitous 'thrush' fungus. Whales, like land mammals, can suffer from skin parasites such as lampreys or infestations of lice that may be the size of a finger-nail, but this was none of their work.

Suddenly I knew what it was that I was looking at. This was frostbite, the scourge of Everest mountaineers, Antartic explorers and naked apes under other circumstances whose skin was exposed for any length of time to sub-zero temperatures. In zoos I'd seen it in young zebras and affecting baboons' tails, but I'd never imagined it could happen in killer whales, creatures of the coldest seas. These were the animals that had apparently flung themselves up onto the ice in pursuit of Scott and his fellow-explorers in the Antarctic, that are feared as 'Lords of the Sea' by the Eskimo hunters of the Canadian Arctic and that themselves go a-hunting after anything that moves in the waters around Greenland. Still, there was no doubt in my mind that frostbite, never before seen in either wild or captive cetaceans, had somehow struck these creatures. I would need to examine the surviving animals to see what could be done and then consider how such a surprising condition had arisen. My 'long johns' would have to wait a bit longer.

Jon drove me back to Saedyrasafnid. I decided to complete my examinations there before discussing the frostbite question with him. The whale pool had been drained down and the three whales now lay on the sandy bottom in about three feet of seawater. Borrowing some fisherman's waders, I climbed down a ladder into the pool and moved among the whales who lay placidly blowing plumes of vapour into the icy evening air. The walls of the almost empty pool sheltered me from the still angry wind, but the chill water quickly made my knees begin to knock as I pored over the animals in the glow from an arc light. I stood by their jaws and bent down to sniff their breath; two had the normal, sweet, cow-like odour, the third was unpleasant. All of them had the same kind of damaged skin that I'd seen in their dead companion. As they flexed their long backs the splits running down to the blubber yawned sickeningly. A killer whale's skin is normally cool, but the thick plaques of tissue on these animals felt unnaturally cold and hard to the touch. What had been living tissue had been frozen to death, converted irreversibly into little more than plastic. The point was, however, that the expanses of killed flesh were still attached to a living body. What would happen next?

I checked the lung and heart sounds with my stethoscope and found that the one with the foul breath had early signs of lung inflammation. Holding a glass plate containing nutrient jelly medium over the blow-hole, I waited for the whale to breathe and blow bacteria onto the plate so that I could have it incubated and examined in the laboratory. Odd, I thought, as I stood with my numb legs pressed to the killer's cheek – not long ago this animal with its four dozen fearsome teeth was out at sea and thought nothing of swimming straight into a great blue whale's mouth and biting a fifty-pound chunk off its victim's tongue, yet here I am with my ankle a tasty morsel for the taking and it doesn't show one iota of aggression or displeasure. Imagine walking up to a tiger or a hyena or a zebra shortly after it had been captured and standing near its head without getting severely 'done'.

To complete my examination I asked Jon and Gunnar to come down and hold the whales' great tail-flukes out of the water so that I could take blood samples. While they put on their waders I checked the sex of the creatures as well as I could by reaching under the water to feel the appropriate bits of anatomy (killer whales are built differently to land mammals and sexing can be very tricky). I have never experienced water so bitterly icy. After fumbling around the genital slits of an animal for a bare thirty seconds, the pain as the cold bit through to the bones of my hand was so acute, and movement of my fingers so difficult, that I had to give up.

Good as gold and quite unlike dolphins, who object to folk with needles, the whales allowed me to draw off my samples without moving their flukes one inch. I had to start treatment of the pneumonic animal right away. I went to my bag for one of the special whale needles and gave an injection of trimethoprim deep into the whale's lumbar muscles. The damaged skin needed heavy application of Dermobion, an ointment only available in Britain. I would telephone Hanne to send several pounds of the stuff out on the next plane. Meanwhile I would make do with a mixture of sulphonamide and ladies' vanishing cream smeared thoroughly into the skin fissures.

'Start filling up the pool. Let's go. I've several things to do,' I said when the whales had been satisfactorily anointed. We climbed up the ladder and Jon turned on the seawater pump.

'Well, Doctor, now tell me what you make of this business.' Jon set down two glasses of brennevin and a plate of hakarl, slivers of raw shark meat that have been buried under shingle for a week or two, look like Parma ham and taste like decomposing dolphin. We were in the Loftleidir Hotel, the best base for me in Iceland. There I could telephone, telex, use the air terminal which is part of the lobby or the airport that adjoins the car park, eat thirty varieties of herring and bathe in the natural hot spring pool in the basement.

'The problem, Jon, is frostbite,' I replied, 'nothing more and nothing less than the disease which you as an Icelandic seaman must be familiar with.'

'But how could that happen? To killer whales that live all their lives in terrible cold seas and the worst weather!'

'If you notice, the damaged areas of skin are all on the upper parts of the whales' bodies — above the waterline, so to speak.'

'That is true.' Jon was looking puzzled.

'There's no doubt in my mind that it's frostbite, but it isn't the cold water that kills the flesh – the animals are able to cope with that – it's the air.'

'How do you mean?'

'Seawater can only get so cold before it freezes solid. In the liquid state it cannot be cold enough to damage the skin of a living, active whale. The animals have a superb heat-exchange system, rather like the central heating in a house, that regulates the temperature of the entire body.'

'But why doesn't frostbite go for wild killer whales north of the Arctic circle? That's where you'll find really cold air.' Jon sipped his glass of fiery spirit and looked even more puzzled.

'Because, Jon, I believe something happened to the whales in the pool at Saedyrasafnid that couldn't have happened in the wild and with which they weren't able to cope.'

'Such as?'

'Well, I've got a shrewd idea, but first let me ask you to tell me about the weather just before the whales developed what you thought was "funny skin".'

Jon sat thinking for some minutes. Then he sent for refills of brennevin and more canapés, this time of dried fish and butter. Presently he began to relate what had happened. The week before the trouble had first been noticed was one of unusually cold weather, the temperatures recorded being the lowest since 1918. Combined with the cold were high winds and falls of snow. Rough seas had damaged the piping that supplied the water to the whale pools, water circulation had broken down and the pool water had become even colder than the ocean nearby.

'Was the whale pool brimming full when all this happened?' I asked.

'Yes, to give the animals maximum water volume.' I was getting a clear picture of the frostbite process now. 'And something happened when the pipes were damaged and pumping stopped that I can't recall seeing before,' Jon continued. 'Snow falling on the pool surface didn't melt but formed a sort of mush on top of the water. It got to be several inches thick except where the whales lay in the centre.'

That was it – the full explanation. 'Didn't anyone break up and disperse the snow mush?' I enquired.

'It happened during the night when no-one was around,' Jon answered. 'Next morning I smashed it.'

Frostbite doesn't occur in the open ocean because the whales are mainly under water, and even when they come up to breathe they stay on the surface for only a short period during which waves will keep the exposed skin wet and relatively 'warm'. Also the activity of the animals probably increases warm blood-flow through the skin. But with Jon's whales there had been a dangerous combination of factors – a brimming pool which exposed the whales to moving streams of ultra-cold air, and a restricted space in the middle of the pool which remained free of mushy snow where the animals in effect had to bask. Their upper parts had dried out in the blast coming off the sea and their skin cells had died just as easily as any other animal's cells will when the protoplasm within them is frozen solid. I explained the process to Jon and we discussed how to avoid such disasters in the future.

'No more brimming pools,' I said. 'Even only a foot or two of wall above the water surface should give some protection from the wind-chill effect. Best of all, build a simple wooden roof.'

The question now was what to do with the three whales. No-one would want to buy them in their present condition and returning them immediately to sea would be grossly irresponsible. We decided to tackle any internal medical problems such as the pneumonia that were probably secondary to the frostbite, patch up the skin and get healing started and then release the animals back to the ocean. Jon took my samples to the Reykjavik hospital for rapid analysis and after calling Hanne with my request for the special ointment, I went and sat in a piping hot spring of sulphurous water near the hotel to ease my still chilled legs, and stared up into the black and windy sky as snowflakes began to fall.

The Dermobion ointment arrived on the next day's plane as arranged but we then ran into difficulties with the Icelandic customs. Urgent consignments, killer whales, sick, for the treatment of, didn't fit into one of their normal categories of imports and it took Jon's son three days to get the medicament released. It is infuriating how bureaucratic customs men of all nationalities can be where livestock is concerned, and the well-being of the animal too often takes second or even third place. Among numerous instances of asinine red tape I have come across was the Spanish guardia who, demanding an official certificate stating that a dolphin had been in its country of origin for three months, refused to accept the appropriate document produced by the animal's attendant which stated that it had been there for ninety days. The cretinous official argued for a whole hour that three months and ninety days are not the same thing and finally sent the poor creature back where it came from, subjecting it to another twelve hours on the road.

Every day I injected the whales and treated their skin, and although each time it took only a few minutes for the cold to strike through to my knees, I still didn't make time to go hunting woollen long johns. The blood samples of the whale with pneumonia gradually improved and the animals began to eat heartily and move more actively in their pool. When the Dermobion finally arrived I applied it deep into the skin splits and protected it with thick lanolin. Massive doses of vitamins were administered via the fish. One of the most important vitamins for marine mammals is thiamine, vitamin B_1. A killer whale the size of these requires about 2000 milligrammes of the chemical every day where a dolphin needs only 300 milligrammes and an adult human a mere 1 milligramme. Deficiency of thiamine causes the tropical disease, beri-beri, something not at all likely to break out in the affluent Icelandic population, so I found it difficult to obtain thiamine tablets for the whales and impossible to locate any containing more than a single milligramme. To avoid giving a daily dosage of 2000 tablets of thiamine as well as the other numerous vitamins, I phoned Marty Dinnes in California and he shipped out some special whale vitamin pills. Again the customs delayed treatment for a few days.

At last, after two weeks of careful medication, I was satisfied that the animals were healthy inside and healing steadily on the surface. The ugly scarring and sloughing on the skin precluded any idea of sending them to a marineland in Europe or the USA. It was time to set them free. One night Jon and his men lowered the water in their pool for the last time, guided the unresisting whales into canvas slings lined with soft woollen blankets and hoisted them out by means of a crane. The slings were placed in large oblong boxes and loaded onto the back of a truck which took them down to the catching-boat waiting in the harbour at Hafnarfjördhur. Jon sailed the boat and its returning cargo of killer whales far out to sea beyond the twenty-mile line and then gently lowered the three into the water. Released from their slings they gave a few powerful strokes of their tail-flukes and dived beyond reach of the ship's searchlight and out of sight.

Next morning the burghers of Hafnarfjördhur awoke to find three killer whales in the harbour, swimming from one fishing-boat to another and begging for food. Although Icelandic fishermen have no great love of the powerful animal that sometimes steals their catches out of the very nets, and have on one notorious occasion in recent years called in the planes of the US Air Force stationed at Keflavik to use the freebooting pods of killer whales as bombing targets, no-one harmed the mendicant trio on this occasion. Some fishermen even tossed the odd bucketful of herring their way.

Jon worriedly brought me the news that raised spectres of the three remaining as permanent scavengers in the port. Had we irrevocably broken the animals' natural ability to hunt for themselves by the weeks of captivity and three-meals-a-day provision of dead fish? It was agreed that Jon should pass the word to everyone in Hafnarfjördhur not to feed a scrap of food to the whales. The next twenty-four hours was tough for some of the softer-hearted folk in Hafnarfjördhur. It was the same as resisting the appealing eyes of your pet dog when he begs for just one chocolate drop or a morsel from your table – but writ large, and in triplicate. The whales rolled on their sides and gazed with one up-turned dark and gleaming eye from which streamed the syrupy tears. They opened pink jaws beneath fishermen mending nets on the jetties and gave appealing piggy squeaks. They followed through the water as men trundled blocks of frozen herring along the quayside. To a man, the citizens of Hafnarfjördhur managed to harden their hearts and resist the temptation to drop a fish accidentally on purpose into the sea.

As darkness fell the three whales were still cruising round the trawlers hollering for a handout, but when the sky lightened late the next morning, they had gone. There was no sign of the animals, nor were they ever sighted again. I like to think that during the night they discussed in their mysterious language of clicks and groans the fickleness of human-kind and then, with the stars bright in the brittle air to navigate by, set out for the Greenland banks where they sensed the great herring shoals would be at that time of year. I must believe that those three whales, carrying the tiny grey scars of my injection sites and the bigger ones where the frostbite healed as only whale-skin can, still swim, and hunt, still leap and dive and sniff the salt air somewhere far from land.

Arriving back from Iceland, I found that the Greenpeace organisation had put out an amount of publicity attacking the taking of killer whales by the Icelanders. They had got many of their facts hopelessly wrong and made much of some photographs which showed my trio of whales after application of the special ointment. The green and white patches of ointment were identified by them as areas of diseased skin. They repeated this mistake several more times, even going so far as to claim that the creamy lanolin mixture which we use to protect the bodies of all healthy cetaceans during transport was frostbite.

We have always tried to avoid clashing with Greenpeace and similar bodies over the question of the small whales and dolphins being exhibited in marinelands and dolphinaria. I can't go along with some of their more extreme members who criticise marine zoos with more and more noise but with surprisingly little scientifically based argument for ammunition. Wild talk about dolphins 'committing suicide after developing psychoses' in captivity is balderdash: although young dolphins can commit

115

suicide by holding their breaths when first caught, Andrew and I do careful autopsies on ninety per cent of cetaceans that die in European pools and we find conclusive physical and pathological causes in every one.

Concerning the plight of the great whales I strongly support the general line of Greenpeace, and just before the Icelandic frostbite case a representative of Greenpeace in London phoned me to ask my opinion of a scheme they were considering adopting against the Japanese whaling fleet. The idea would be to use dart-rifles to shoot syringes containing radio-active isotopes into a whale after it had been harpooned by the whalers. Radio-active contamination of the carcass of the whale would render it unsaleable and also constitute a powerful symbolic gesture to the nation that, along with the Russians, wreaks the most serious and irresponsible havoc among the diminishing herds of these stupendous animals. Greenpeace were also interested in the possibility of darting pain-killers or euthanasing drugs into dying harpooned whales.

Parts of their proposals appealed to me. I didn't like the isotope bit and could see innumerable problems, but I suggested that female sex hormone might make an equally good and cheap alternative. Remembering the fuss that there had been a few years earlier in Germany and the USA when the rumour went round that the practice of caponising chickens and enhancing their growth by the implantation of oestrogen pellets in their necks might be having a feminising effect on virile males who ate the chicken meat, I could imagine a bit of shrewd PR combined with the injection of a few whales causing similar consternation among the Japanese public. Once darted into a whale, the stable oestrogen chemicals couldn't be neutralised, washed or cooked out. As for the admirably humane suggestion of relieving the suffering of a whale dying, as they do, with a thing shaped like a small anchor with a hand-grenade stuck on the end exploded in its belly, I couldn't help. There just isn't any drug that is sufficiently fast-acting, as well as being safe to handle and capable of having a dose big enough for a whale concentrated into the volume of the largest syringe that a dart-gun can fire (20 ccs). Such a drug may come in time, of course, and perhaps then we may read of the *Rainbow Warrior* sailing into battle, its decks lined with dart-gun-toting marksmen.

I also found when I got back to England that I couldn't shake off the ache in my knees, and what felt like crunchy gravel had made an appearance over my knee-caps. Hanne was furious when she found out that I had never bought the long johns, and my osteopath diagnosed chronically inflamed joints that were certain to stay as a permanent reminder of the first, and I hope last, case of frostbite to be seen in killer whales.

I hadn't been home twenty-four hours when all thoughts about whales of any type were displaced by other pressing matters, this time on terra firma. As I drove back from my delayed routine visit to the zoo at Chessington, Liliana came through on the radio-telephone from Madrid. Chang-Chang, the male panda there, had collapsed and was semi-conscious. Would I go out straightaway?

I pulled up in a farm gateway on the Oxshott road and referred to my ABC airlines timetable. The next BA flight to Madrid took off in an hour. I set off again and made for Heathrow. On the way I put through a call to Hanne, who by now was accustomed to a permanently unpredictable life. Cancelling a dinner appointment with friends on one occasion isn't difficult but when one does it again a second time to the same people, perhaps giving them so little notice that it's impossible to make alternative arrangements, I often wonder whether our guests accept an apologetic 'David's in Spain with a panda' or 'He's got a hippo bad but may be back next week' at face value or secretly investigate the possibility that they've contracted BO. Hanne coped well. A fine cook in the German style, her pots of sauerkraut mit speck and sorrel soup don't spoil and indeed improve with keeping the odd day or two. She handled awkward changes of plans with equanimity and when holding the fort by telephone relished the regular opportunity to converse with clients in her native tongue. After English, German is unquestionably the most important language in our work with exotic creatures. It is the lingua franca of many zoos behind the Iron Curtain, German, Austrian and Swiss directors run parks across the world from Arabia to Latin America and for Andrew and me Germany, the country possessing the most top-quality zoos in Europe, is as busy a part of our practice as Great Britain.

I caught the Madrid flight in the nick of time and sat back over a cup of coffee to consider Liliana's brief message. Collapsed and semi-conscious, she had said. Curious, I thought, how I never ever hear things like that reported about lions or bears. Commoner animals do seem to get commoner complaints, but rare animals like to make life difficult. Should anyone ever succeed in nabbing the Loch Ness Monster and exhibiting it in the Highland Wildlife Park at Kingussie, I bet my bottom dollar that the first time it falls sick it will be with a funny-looking disease caused by a little-known germ that is described as producing attacks of flatulence in a particular tribe of pygmies in the Umbagumba River region of the Congo and is resistant to all known drugs. No way will it get a streptococcal sore throat that responds dramatically to a penicillin lozenge administered in whatever Nessie feeds on. The Gods don't smile on horse-doctors.

Certainly I was absolutely in the dark over Chang-Chang. I could only hope that whatever had caused the collapse, it wasn't the heart or some sort of crisis in the brain. Just my luck, I thought – the first emergency with a giant panda and it might be my last.

The two-hour flight felt like two days. I was first off the plane and through passports and customs. Thank God taxis are like flies round a midden at Madrid airport with none of the queueing and extortion of J. F. Kennedy in New York or the chicanery of Heathrow. Twenty-five minutes after I landed I was across the city and going into the zoo. Fearful that I might be too late, I jogged through the grounds to the panda house. Everyone who had anything to do with the pandas was there, gathered in the little kitchen. I looked at their faces straightaway; you can see at a glance whether the worst has happened. They all looked morose but relieved to see me in the same moment. There was none of the familiar expressions of resignation that signify a death. Chang-Chang was still alive. Tenser than usual under such circumstances, I cut out the pleasantries and asked at once how he was.

Dr Celma, the biological director of the zoo, answered. 'He sleeps deeply all the time,' she said. 'He rouses a little occasionally but soon relapses. He hasn't eaten for twenty-four hours.'

I peeped through the observation window in the door to Chang-Chang's sleeping quarters. He lay on his wooden bed-shelf, a motionless heap of harlequin fur that might have been one of the expensive life-size panda toys or pyjama-cases that Harrods stock at Christmas. 'Can I go in?' I asked Antonio-Luis who knew the animal best, having brought the pandas from China along with key words in Chinese panda-talk to make them feel at home.

'Certainly, and I think you will be able to touch him if you wish. He sleeps muy profundo – very deeply.'

I cautiously opened the door and went in. Not only was the panda sleeping very much profundo, he was actually snoring. I reached out and gently touched his rump. There was no reaction but I glanced round to make sure that my escape route was clear if Chang-Chang should suddenly come to; I had been bitten once by a jaguar that was 'definitely in a deep coma for the last couple of days, Doctor, honest!' in a similar situation. I worked my hand slowly under the warm thigh to feel for the femoral artery and found it exactly where it lies on more mundane creatures. So pandas are orthodox in at least one respect, I thought. The pulse was strong and regular. I tapped the panda on his belly; he gave a deep sigh and snored on. Moving up to his head, I pulled out my stethoscope and pressed the diaphragm against his chest wall. As I listened to my first panda heart sounds and the soft swish of the lungs, everything seemed normal. His ears were cool to the touch and flicked when I tickled inside them, so he wasn't too deeply unconscious. Very gently, but with a strong feeling of excitement, I began stroking his neck and slowly inched my hand upwards to his cheek. When I reached the lips I delicately folded back first the upper and then the lower one; the colour was a satisfactory pale pink. I prodded the abdomen, but it was relaxed and I couldn't feel any lumps or areas of tension. There was just one more thing I wanted to do. Taking out my thermometer, I lubricated it with a blob of saliva and went to his rear end. If anything could disturb his unnatural slumber it might be this. I slipped the little bulb of mercury into Chang-Chang's rectum. He was totally oblivious. A minute later I read his temperature – 39°C. That was probably OK, but at that time no-one knew the correct normal body temperature of the giant panda, for pandas aren't the sort of creatures to take lightly to having things inserted into their nether regions when they're hale and hearty.

Apart from the state of insensibility there wasn't anything out of the ordinary, but what is ordinary in a beast of this sort?

'Any diarrhoea, vomiting, anything else unusual?' I asked Liliana.

'Nothing.'

'And he fed and behaved normally up until a day ago?'

'Yes.'

It was just as I had feared. I hadn't got any idea as to the nature of the strange somnolence. 'But are you sure that there was nothing new added to the diet, no fresh batch of bamboo?'

'No, absolutamente no.'

I asked to see the daily diary kept by the panda keepers. A meticulous record of food consumption, body weight, environmental and climatic conditions, it might conceivably give some clue, perhaps to food-poisoning or some allergic reaction. I went back to the page dated a week previously and then began turning the pages slowly. Columns of neat figures. Litres of milk. Kilos of bamboo, cereals and fruit. In the 'Comments' section the occasional entry: 'Weather too hot – preferred to stay in the shade'; or 'Very active between 10 am and noon'. Nothing significant. Then I reached the entries for the last forty-eight hours. The menus for the two animals and their appetites had been the same as ever, it appeared, but I saw three words tacked onto the usual list of foodstuffs. I struggled to decipher the handwriting – pastillas contra lombrices, that was it, tablets against worms.

'What's this?' I asked. 'Worm tablets?'

Liliana nodded. 'Oh, yes, I forgot to tell you. We gave some anti-worm drugs.'

'Why?'

120

'The panda keeper found a worm in the droppings of one of the animals.'

'Are you sure it was a parasitic worm, not one from the grass in the paddock?' I had examined samples of the pandas' stools which I'd taken back to England after my first visit to them. Not a single parasite could I or the laboratory at Weybridge find.

'We decided to play safe. We gave one dose of piperazine in the food.'

Liliana showed me the bottle of piperazine tablets, the ones commonly used in every country against worms of dogs and cats. The dose had been a stiff one, enough for a Great Dane of the same weight. I began to wonder. Piperazine has been used in domestic animals for years with excellent results. I couln't recall a single case of trouble other than the occasional individual who brought the stuff back up, and I'd dispensed literally hundredweights of it. The veterinary reference books classified it as of low toxicity with ill effects, even from overdosage, unlikely. But for some time I'd had an ill-defined sense of unease about piperazine in certain exotic species. Matt Kelly had reported to me that lions which I'd dosed with it at Belle Vue had been 'drunk' for twenty-four hours after. At the time I'd been sceptical of Matt's story, and I hadn't been able to reproduce the 'drunken lion' effect in big cats in circuses who were and remain enthusiastic users of the drug. More ominously I'd heard, but been unable to track down the source of the statement, that piperazine had actually killed adult lions. There were warnings of possible trouble in sealions also coming from the United States and I knew that overdosage in human beings affected the nervous system.

I was sure that I'd hit upon the cause of Chang-Chang's stupor. One of the many little differences about pandas, it would seem, was an intolerance to piperazine. Now I had to consider treatment. Nothing specific would neutralise piperazine. The reference book that I carry in the Bag wasn't any help and a call to England to the Poison Bureau that is manned round the clock at Guy's Hospital resulted, once the doctor on duty had been persuaded that talk of panda intoxication wasn't a joke, in general advice to keep body systems supported by any means available.

Shao-Shao, the female panda, who had received the same dose of the wormer, was completely unaffected. Perhaps Chang-Chang was peculiarly sensitive to the chemical or had a liver that had trouble in getting rid of it. I decided to go for the liver theory and at the same time give the brain and nervous system a boost by injecting a massive dose of vitamin B. I loaded a syringe with the golden-brown liquid that smells like Marmite and gave the shot into the slumbering panda's leg. 'Nothing more,' I said. 'Just an alert watch through the night.' We all looked glum.

After discussing my opinion with the Spaniards, we dispersed except for Antonio-Luis and one of the panda keepers who would maintain a vigil over the patient. The tension would persist until it became clear which way Chang-Chang was going to go. I felt tired and on edge. No promenade down the Paseo de la Castellana this evening. I would go straight to my hotel, phone Andrew if I could locate him – discussing the case with him would ease things – and then try to get to sleep. I would be back at the panda house at the crack of dawn. St Francis of Assisi, ora pro nobis.

As the first chink of grey light silhouetted the city skyline of apartment blocks with their curiously passé style and window-boxes like the hanging gardens of Babylon, I returned to the Casa de Campo. The little groups of young aficionados with their matadors' cloaks and sets of bull's horns were already gathering under the trees to practise their veronicas and faroles in bloodless imitation of their heroes of the Plaza de Toros. Inside the zoo cranes and pelicans strode round the silent pathways, looking at the displays as if with the interest of early-rising natural history students, and the nosey-parker prairie dogs busied themselves officiously on the door-steps of their burrows in the lawns. Early morning is the best time to go round any zoo. With no need to put on airs and graces for the rubber-necking primates on the other side of the wire or moat, the animals appear distinctly more natural. The poseurs and dandies and wallflower-types can relax before the ungainly herd of visitors is let in.

I'd have been telephoned at my hotel if Chang-Chang's condition had deteriorated. Even so I felt apprehensive as I squelched through the disinfectant foot-bath at the entrance to the panda house. 'Buenos dias,' I called as I hurried down the dark passageway. I sounded remarkably cheerful.

Antonio-Luis stuck his red-eyed face out of the kitchen door. He gave a fatigued but still radiant smile. 'Muy buenos dias, David. Todo esta bien – all is well. Chang-Chang is awake. Listen!'

I stopped for a moment. There was a querulous mewing sound coming from behind the male panda's door. I darted to the peep-hole. Chang-Chang was pacing irritably about his bedroom, plainly disgusted by the delay in serving breakfast.

'Mo-mo. Mo-mo.' I cooed the Chinese words that Antonio-Luis had told me were appropriate on such occasions. The panda looked up, bright-eyed and expectant, and I felt a rush of exhilaration. He was going to be all right.

When the large dish of milk, egg and porridge had been rustled up I gave the word for it to be given to Chang-Chang. Quick as a flash he scoffed the lot and came mewing back for more. Whether the injection had played a part in his recovery or not we would never know. It may have been spontaneous wearing-off of the effects of the piperazine. But what did it really matter! We had come through our first brush with sickness in the giant panda unscathed.

I was pleased as Punch as I packed up my things to return to London, but before leaving I made a cast-iron arrangement with my Spanish colleagues: in future not a single tablet or teaspoonful of any sort of nostrum, medicament or elixir, not even half an aspirin, would be given to the pandas without contacting me first. 'Don't forget that penicillin is lethal for the humble guinea-pig,' I reminded them. 'Who knows what dangerous idiosyncratic reactions might lie in wait for us in pandas in the future. Next time we may not be so lucky.'

7

Wild animals are not always as clean, cuddly or aesthetically pleasing as many of the less well-informed visitors to zoos and wildlife parks might wish. In fact, I have often wondered whether it would not be sensible to educate the public in unfamiliar aspects of exotic biology by erecting some sort of notice at appropriate times. Antelopes that trail a rope of placenta for some hours after calving and the hippos that sometimes produce red perspiration and appear to be literally sweating blood are common causes of complaints by visitors. I am totally against any suggestion that animals living their normal lives should be taken off exhibition at times like these: humans must see the beasts, imagined warts and all. That goes for mating animals, too. Most zoo directors have had letters or phone calls from people who thought that it was most improper for the zebras or the monkeys or the lions to be allowed to copulate in public, particularly when there were children around. Ah, well, I used to say, you try stopping some of the zebras, monkeys and lions that I know.

The other side of the coin is the inordinate fascination that the coupling of great beasts has for some folk. At Belle Vue the aquatic love-making of the hippos always drew crowds of middle-aged ladies who generally feigned ignorance as to what was going on but stayed all afternoon by the hippo pool watching the 'charming games'. The lone male visitors in dirty raincoats preferred the performance of the rather well-blessed male tapir or the winsome little wanderoo monkey that had an eye for ladies with good figures, would beckon appealingly to them and, when they reached out a hand over the barrier to touch the sweet little thing, would do things in the twinkling of an eye that would have had him in court and on the front page of the *News of the World* if he'd been on the other side of the bars. Most bizarre of all was the man who for at least five years brought his lunch to the monkey house each day to watch the same one o'clock porno show put on by the mandrills. I swear the monkeys waited until the chap got into place and unwrapped his sandwiches before beginning.

Although I contend that humans must be encouraged to see the whole range of normal animal behaviour, there are certain obvious exceptions such as when cheetahs need privacy in order to pluck up the nerve to mate or when, with some species, birth is imminent. It was idiotic, for example, when the zoo in Mexico City allowed people to take photographs of their new-born giant panda; as I predicted, it didn't survive beyond a few days. Animals that are sick or have undergone surgical operations sometimes need to be kept away from the gawking public. On other occasions, again ideally with an explanatory notice provided, visitors should see with their own eyes the care and skill employed by the zoo and its veterinary services in keeping wild animals fit and healthy. They need reminding that animals like humans can and do suffer from disease. Earlier in my career, while I was still based in the North, the then director at Belle Vue, Ray Legge, and I had had a brush with the RSPCA over this.

It was a foul-weathered Saturday night with incessant heavy rain and wind. I was snug in my favourite room, the one with mullioned windows on three sides, in the old farmhouse outside Rochdale, lying flat on the floor with Vivaldi at full volume and Lupin the cat snoozing deeply on my cheek, when the telephone rang by my side. It was Ray and he sounded alarmed. 'Had a call from security to check the paddock house for the usual Saturday night vandals,' he explained in his precise, rather military style. 'Went past the deer range and heard some sort of ruckus among the Père Davids. I had a look as best I could with a torch in this confounded weather and saw what looks like an eye knocked out!'

'Give me thirty minutes. I'll meet you at the deer range.' I peeled off the dreaming cat and got up to go for my coat.

It cannot be said too often that veterinary medicine, of exotic animals in particular, is no profession for devotees of James Herriot, for the children of doting parents whose letters to me always stress how their Johnny or Jane just adored helping the farmer next door bottle-feed his early lambs or did so marvellously well grooming guinea-pigs for the local show. Veterinary medicine isn't 'Animal Magic' crossed with 'Dr Kildare'. It has much more in common with the blood and guts and pain of front-line battlefield surgery. For me a good vet has to be filled with the magic of the disease process. He has to live in a world of miraculous and intricate machines that are preyed upon by invisible but mighty assailants – viruses, strange germs, molecules that can poison, enfeeble or block vital processes, and mysterious keys and talismans that still wait to be discovered. The world within these living machines, the complexity and cleverness of the pus cell, the power at the command of one single infinitesimally small but tortured neuron, the ebb and flow of a multitude of cunning fluids, and the all-pervading cycle of life and death – here is his workshop. Shattered bone struggling to mend, pain grimly borne by animals without the inclination to scream, a world of creatures that don't look at life and suffering as we humans do – that's what it's all about. Stroking puppies and slapping show ponies is just the froth.

Talk of eye injuries, for example, often makes folk feel queasy. The eye is thought of as a delicate and fragile bubble. Certainly it is a most subtly constructed organ, the only part of the brain in fact which is permanently on view, but it is also amazingly tough and resilient. I'd learned when I first began to take a special interest in the surgery of the eye that one could set about it with scalpels, forceps and silken sutures in much the same way as other parts of the body; it wasn't a balloon that popped and disappeared as soon as you touched it. I also knew that in most cases where the eye was knocked out and remained attached, the vital nerve and the muscles which control movement of the eyeball are stretched but still remain intact. I'd had dozens of animals in that condition and very few had lost their sight, provided action had been taken immediately.

126

Eyes knocked out of Père David deer are not for the squeamish. Most people have heard how this swamp-loving animal, originally of China, Manchuria and Japan and once thought to be extinct, was discovered in 1865 to be surviving still in the walled hunting-park of the Chinese emperor by the French priest who gave the species its name. Unlike other deer it has a long tail and antlers with long forks and no tines over the brows. It also has very protuberant eyes that give it a strange, inquisitive look. As with Pekinese dogs and some species of sealion who also possess bulging eyes, it occasionally happens that a blow can dislocate the eye out of its socket in the skull.

That Saturday night, Ray and I stood in the darkness and driving rain in front of the Père David enclosure and played the beam of a torch on the stag in question. It had been squabbling in the rain with one of its companions and a chance flick of the antlers had caught the left eye, which now lay grotesquely outside the lower eyelid but thankfully still attached.

'We'll need to put it out straightaway,' I said. 'There's a fair chance of saving the vision in the eye. Do we have any staff about?'

Ray shook his head. Matt Kelly was out and Len, and assistant head keeper, was ill in bed.

'Right. We can do it ourselves. I'll get the gun ready. Could you get a bottle of liquid paraffin from the medical cupboard, please?'

Ray squelched off through the downpour and I took shelter in my car to make up the little aluminium dart with its needle, plunger and explosive charge. When it was assembled I filled it with the powerful anaesthetic drug, etorphine, breaking the rules because I was alone. I'd used etorphine, or M99 as it was originally known, ever since it had first been developed by Reckitt and Colman, the drug company better known for the mustard they manufacture. In those days I'd helped in the first studies of the effects of the new wonder drug on exotic species. We had found that it was superb for zebras, gazelles, gnu and oryx, that elephants and rhinos were super-sensitive to it, that it turned tigers and lions into raving maniacs, tended to kill monkeys, make buffaloes randy and yaks vomit, and didn't seem to dope crocodiles very much at all. I had happily handled large quantities of the crystalline chemical during the anaesthesia of hundreds of animals from bears to bison. It turned out to be the best contribution to zoo animal medicine ever discovered.

Unfortunately, it soon became obvious that while it was safe for many species of animals it was incredibly dangerous to primates, including man. When veterinary surgeons started to die through accidentally coming into contact with surprisingly tiny amounts of the stuff and when others found it a fast and pleasant means of suicide, everyone became very much aware of etorphine's awesome power even in microscopical amounts. Worse, it seemed that it could pass through the membranes of the eye, nose and mouth and through invisible abrasions on the skin. Junkies in America quickly discovered the potential of the drug and for a short time we feared that it would be completely withdrawn from manufacture in Great Britain. Happily this didn't come to pass but, apart from the statutory narcotics control to which it was quite properly subjected, conventions for handling the chemical came into use. The special antidote to the anaesthetic, different from the one which reverses the effect in animals, is always carried in the bag along with the etorphine. Most vets use the so-called 'buddy' system, never touching etorphine without having a colleague present ready to jab them with the antidote should a needle slip or some liquid spill, accidents which can easily happen when working among animals. Years ago, before all the fuss, I'd handled etorphine with confidence; now, constantly reminded of the risks we were taking in handling it, my fingers seemed to tremble as I drew the golden liquid from the bottle and ironically made the likelihood of a miscalculation more possible. I'd told people like Ray Legge and others with whom I regularly worked where I carried the antidote and how to stick it straight through the seat of my pants and into my buttocks without going through any formalities should they find me going woozy on them. So, with etorphine capable of killing a man within minutes, I was taking a chance that night by filling the syringe with Ray gone and nobody around.

128

When Ray returned with the liquid paraffin I took the torch and stood close to the fence of the Père David enclosure. It wouldn't have been wise to go in at that point; these deer, and especially the stags, were mean-tempered and dangerous. I aimed the dart-gun down the line of the torch-beam and, when a suitable expanse of shoulder muscle was illuminated, I made allowance for the sweep of the wind and rain and pulled the trigger. The dart flashed in the yellow glow and I heard it thwack home and softly explode. Ray and I sat in the car for the three minutes it took for the stag to collapse unconscious.

The rain increased its ferocity as we went into the enclosure and Ray armed himself with a stick to beat off any of the other deer which might intrude upon the al fresco operating site. Nothing intrigues animals as much as one of their number behaving strangely under the influence of drugs; even domestic cattle gather in rapt amazement around one of their fellows lying anaesthetised in a field. With wild animals, their instinctive distrust of anything that is out of the ordinary in their environment can lead them to attack en masse a sedated or unconscious individual. I knelt down in the mud and began to work by torchlight.

It was miserable in every way. The rain whipped across my eyes and spattered mud onto the deer's face. Sterility was out of the question. Unprepared by a few hours of fasting for general anaesthetic, the animal began to regurgitate its stomach contents. A soup of water and half-digested vegetation streamed out of its nostrils. I wiped them clear in the fading little circle of light from the torch, knowing that I would have to work fast to avoid losing the patient from self-drowning. I heard Ray curse in the darkness as one of the other stags took a swing at him.

With slipping fingers I unscrewed the top of the bottle and splashed liquid paraffin liberally over the deer's dislocated eye and its face all around. Then I began gently wiping blood and mud and dirt from the inflamed cornea of the eye. When the major bits of filth had been removed I put the torch into my mouth and held it between my teeth, directing the light onto the eyeball. With both hands I cupped the eye and began to exert firm, even pressure. I remembered the first time I'd replaced an eye: a Peke belonging to a swine of a breeder who didn't like young vets, had halitosis and never did pay the 8/6 fee for the operation. 'God, make it go back,' I prayed as I pressed harder towards the socket and the water ran down the back of my neck and my knees sank deeper in the mud.

Suddenly, as should happen, the eye plopped into its rightful hole in the skull with a 'thwuck' that I could hear through my fingers. 'It's in,' I shouted through the wind.

'Top-hole,' came Ray's reply. 'I don't think I can hold these blighters off much longer.' I heard the twack of his stick against horny antlers.

Now I squirted liberal quantities of an anaesthetic-antibiotic cream onto the eyeball and began stitching the upper and lower eyelids together with nylon. My teeth were aching from gripping the metal torch. When the eye was securely closed I injected tetracyline into the deer's haunch muscle and asked Ray to give me a hand in administering the antidote that should have the animal on its feet within a couple of minutes. Ray crouched beside me, half-turned with one fist jammed into the base of the deer's throat to raise its jugular vein for my injection and the other clasping the stick in case of attack. He kept up a barrage of shouts to deter the deer hidden in the darkness: 'Go on! Gerroutofit! Gertcha!'

The vein didn't appear. I groped in the hair of the neck for the familiar feel of the blood vessel. The torch's light was by now a feeble orange. 'Press lower down and harder!' Together we struggled in the mud. A deer trotted past and sprayed us with more water and dirt. I began to sweat. Suppose I couldn't find the vein, well, there was always the slow route by intramuscular injection – second-best but better than nothing.

Ray gave a yell. 'Dammit, something's just prodded me up my bottom!' He flailed with his stick. 'Go on! Gerrout!' His balled fist shifted its position on the deer's neck and all at once I felt the jugular vibrating under my fingers.

'Got it!' I shouted, and jabbed with the syringe containing the antidote. When it was all in I jumped up. 'Come on, let's get out

130

of here,' I said. When animals come round from etorphine they do it rapidly and completely with no gradual awakening and no dizzy after-effects. It's best to get out of the way as soon as the antidote is in to avoid finding yourself in trouble with a dangerous animal that only a few minutes before was an innocuous an uncaring patient.

A few seconds after the antidote reached the deer's brain, it gave a deep breath, coughed to clear its throat of regurgitated stomach contents and leapt to its feet. We watched it walk steadily out of the flickering torchlight, then Ray and I drove back to his bungalow for coffee and whisky and hot showers.

Next day I went back to Manchester to look at the Père David. I was well satisfied. The eyelids weren't too swollen under the stitches and the animal was otherwise behaving normally. I don't suppose one in a thousand of the visitors noticed the deer with the Nelson look. After three more days I anaesthetised the deer again and took out the sutures. The eyelids opened and there was the eye in its proper place. I squinted through my ophthalmoscope; the surroundings were somewhat bruised and the cornea had been scuffed but the deeper parts of the eye, the iris, lens and retina, appeared in good shape. The pupil reacted to light and I was certain the eye could see. To keep up the antibiotic treatment I injected a small dose of penicillin under the conjunctiva and squeezed in more anaesthetic ointment. The prognosis could not have been better; the animal would be as good as new except for a scar on the cornea that might persist for a few months but wouldn't significantly hinder vision. So it proved: some weeks later the deer did indeed still display a white scar on its eye, the only sign of its accident that stormy evening, but we could see from the way it eyed the females that it hadn't got a blind side.

One morning Ray opened his post to find a strongly worded complaint from the veterinary surgeon who was head of the RSPCA's wildlife department. It appeared that he had visited Belle Vue incognito and had spotted the Père David with the scarred eye. Without taking the matter up with the director or even requesting information, he had returned to his headquarters and attacked the zoo for having an animal with eye disease on display.

I have rarely been more angry. If the fellow had only taken the trouble to telephone Ray or me to ask whether the deer was under treatment, we wouldn't have minded at all. But after a sodden struggle in the dark of a Saturday evening to save an animal's sight and an outcome that was almost perfect, to receive such a missive was decidedly galling. I spent a good hour on the phone inserting the biggest flea I could find into the RSPCA vet's ear. But I come back to the idea that perhaps it is up to us, even with such post-operative cases, to erect some sort of notice. The only question is what it should say. What about 'The management regrets any inconvenience while the animals are under repair?'

In 1979 Andrew and I decided to take a big gamble by employing our first assistant specifically to be resident in the Middle East and based at the large National Zoo of Abu Dhabi at Al Ain. Finding the right guy proved not to be easy. There is no shortage of veterinarians who would like to work with exotic animals, but training them is the first major problem. Some university veterinary faculties give absolutely no instruction on wild animal medicine to undergraduates. The most is provided by Cambridge – a total of one day's lectures in a six-year course. Experienced as a young vet may be in performing Caesarians on sheep or nerve-blocking ponies, how do you let him loose on his first giraffe? Then there are a multitude of other special requirements for the horse-doctor turned lion-leech, especially our globe-trotting variety. In general practice with farmers, dog-breeders and doting cat-fanciers, the treatment of the owner is a more important part of the art of medicine than actually physicking their animals. With the right bed-side, or stable-side, manner I suspect a veterinary surgeon might prosper and gain an enviable reputation even though he lost all his cases. In exotic animal medicine, on the other hand, results count just as much as diplomacy.

The man we needed, in short, was a paragon who would approach the care of everything from monkeys to manatees with the same enthusiasm that Andrew and I shared, would be prepared to work often alone with improvised or even no equipment, would

132

handle Arabs, Levantines, Greeks, Spaniards, Africans, Latins and Teutons with sensitivity, would go at the drop of a hat in the middle of the night to dissect a stranded whale, would possess a constitution that could cope with Bedou food, Suntory whisky, flies, quaint plumbing and the labyrinthine politics that underpin the zoo world, would learn enough of a foreign language or two to know when the man helping him catch the antelope called him 'a bloody foreigner' in his own tongue, and last but not least would push ahead bit by bit each day in the vast virgin fields of zoo medicine.

We spent a long time looking, but then were lucky in finding just such a chap. Chris Furley came to our interview in London wearing one brown and one black sock. He had been brought up mainly in Africa, was a keen linguist and had as his hobbies modern literature and butterfly collecting. He liked simple food which he preferred to cook for himself and he was anxious to start skin-diving. Interestingly, although his experience of zoo medicine had been limited to a period seeing practice at Whipsnade Park, he knew the difference between a Dorcas and a Rhim gazelle when asked, which was more than the rest of our interviewees did. We liked his catholic tastes and his lack of the tunnel-visioned scientist attitude that the universities rejoice in churning out. Andrew appreciated his ordered mind – Chris had catalogued Edinburgh University's collection of lepidoptera – I was impressed by the potted critique of Herman Hesse's writing that he gave me and tickled by the odd socks, and Hanne, who took notes during the interviews, gave him the thumbs-up because of his good German which he had learned while working in Germany for a year after qualifying.

Our selection of Chris as assistant proved justified. He settled down to the job of resident veterinary officer at Al Ain with gusto. Every couple of months Andrew or I would fly down to spend a week with him and we kept up daily contact by phone and telex.

Chris took with him to Abu Dhabi a new model of dart-gun which Andrew and I hoped would provide the happy medium between the short-range, low-powered pistols and the long-range rifles whose power could be altered only by changing the strength of the blank cartridge that operated them − not an easy thing to do when stalking a nervous and fleet-footed target at a constantly varying distance. Hitting flesh with syringes blasted out of these weapons at too close a range could produce alarming results. Even though the needles are fitted with a collar to control depth of penetration, they sometimes weren't able to stop the body of the syringe itself punching out a disc of skin half an inch in diameter. We had never had any fatalities or even complications from this kind of occasional mishap but we knew of cases such as a zebra which was darted with a perfect shot at theoretically reasonable range with a heavy, 15-cc syringe. The syringe had hit the target area on the right haunch and then gone on to travel through the buttock muscle, entered through the archway of the pelvis and finally come to rest in the animal's rectum. Not funny. These weapons are for life-saving, not life-taking.

Now a Liverpool firm had brought out a new and highly successful dart-rifle. The Conservator gun is brilliantly designed and, although also powered by powder charges, its range can be controlled instantly by a wheel on one side of the back-sight. My own first use of it came when a deer escaped from the Anchor Inn zoo (yes, a pub with a surprisingly sizeable collection of exotics in its gardens, including camels) at Gargrave in Yorkshire. The fugitive trooped into the shippon with a herd of cows that it had adopted on a farm some eight miles away when they went home at milking time. After the surprised farmer had finished milking (he didn't try the deer), he let the cows out to pasture again and I sedated the runaway with the Conservator at close range through a hole in the shippon window. The rifle did a splendid job.

On the way back from Gargrave to our northern office in Keighley I stopped in Ilkley where Shelagh, who had remarried, and my daughters were now living. Stephanie, the elder, had begun at Medical School in London but Lindsey, soon to continue her journalistic studies in Birmingham, and Shelagh joined me for dinner at one of the fashionable little town's restaurants, and then I drove on to stay overnight with Andrew and Linda at their home beside the Worth Valley steam railway.

It was another Linda, this time a sea elephant named after the blue-film star, Linda Lovelace, because of her ability to swallow large numbers of Mediterranean mackerel, who indirectly that same week led to me being clobbered by, of all things, a fish. The fish was a gunmetal-blue grouper weighing a mere two kilos, which is nothing for such sea bass which can reach a quarter of a tonne or more. It swam up to the surface, gave sufficient throttle on its tail-fin to lift its snub nose out of the water and smartly bit a generous chunk out of my right index finger. I snatched my hand back, with gore streaming down my trousers and stunned with surprise at the unprovoked attack. It was as if I had been suddenly savaged by a rabbit-punching rabbit or butted in the solar plexus by a rampant duck. Unless one has battled beneath the waves with a shark or barracuda there is surely something less than macho in displaying the scars of such a wound to one's friends and explaining, 'It was a fish wot did it.'

Anyway, I wasn't hunting the great white shark off the Barrier Reef, but rather standing in the back of the Porto Cristo aquarium, Majorca, with Robert Bennett, the new director of the island's marineland, and with nothing further from my mind than submarine adventure. Robert had recently purchased the sea elephant, Linda, and rightly suspecting her to be pregnant, had asked me to go out and check her over. When Linda's pre-natal was finished we had driven to Porto Cristo to look at the problem fish that Robert had been asked to help with. The grouper had one eye that bulged grotesquely from the pressure of the tumour which was destroying it. The sight on that side had gone and to get my finger the fish had turned in the water and lined up his good eye before launching the attack.

'Ho, ho! Incredible!' chortled the Spanish aquarium director who was showing us the sick fish as I staunched the outward and visible sign of yet another of the zoo vet's unsuspected occupational hazards. 'Is cheeky boy, no? Is comico, yes? Me forgettin' to tell you no' to put fingers near Panchito's tank. Don' like strangers.' His stomach wobbled as he giggled uncontrollably. Panchito swam po-faced round his glass-fronted domain and kept the one eye open for further trespassing.

The malignant melanoma tumour had been blooming in Panchito's orbital cavity for several months. The aquarium had bought the grouper years before when he was thumbnail-size. He was by now a fine specimen, the diseased eye excepted, and as he was the oldest inhabitant of the tanks and much respected by the staff who knew when to keep their hands to themselves, no-one wanted to see him taken out as crab-bait.

Although in Belle Vue's heyday the zoo had possessed one of the best aquaria in Great Britain and I had on occasion supplied drugs for the treatment of sick fish, it had always been with the guidance of Ray Legge, the then director and an expert aquarist in his own right. I knew, and know, little about finny matters unless it comes to appreciating a good bouillabaise, Harry Ramsden's famous fish and chips or the green herring that is sold with chopped raw onion from Amsterdam street stalls. Fish, like poultry, are usually in need of mass medication, since their diseases are principally those of the group or shoal. Diagnosis is by sample autopsies. The individual is rarely important or valuable, and his individuality is lost in the consideration of the economics of group therapy and disease control en masse. That's why I've never been interested in poultry or fish medicine. I like individual patients – single characters to wrestle with where the autopsy, although always valuable, comes if it comes at all after doing battle with the disease.

Panchito, however, was quite plainly a singular character and his problems needed the same approach that I would use on a chimp or a Père David deer. 'That eye will have to come out,' I said.

''E will fight when we try to catch him, sin duda. 'E will be muy dificil to hold still under the knife, señor.'

'We're not doing it without anaesthetic, my friend. Fish he may be but he still feels pain.'

Anaesthetising fish is very easy nowadays. It can be done by injection, but usually the sleep-inducing chemical is simply added to the water. The drugs used are not the same as those employed in mammals and birds for general anaesthesia. What I generally prescribe for fish surgery or to sedate them for catching is benzocaine, a human local anaesthetic commonly found as an ingredient of sore-throat lozenges and mouth-ulcer sprays.

After making a calculation of the volume of water in Panchito's tank, I dropped the appropriate quantity of benzocaine crystals into the water – keeping my fingers well clear. Ten minutes later the bellicose grouper lay unconscious on the bottom, gill flaps gently pumping. Robert fished him out with a scoop net and we laid him, bad eye up, on a marble slab. The aquarium director kept the fish wet by spraying him with seawater while Robert held him firmly. I had about ten minutes before he began to come round. It took me about thirty seconds to disinfect the site with mercurochrome and then sweep round the cancerous mass with a stiletto-shaped scalpel. Taking care to leave a safe margin of healthy tissue, I dissected out the eye and plugged the plum-sized hole with gauze. There was little bleeding and no need for forceps. When I was satisfied that I had left behind no scraps of malignant tissue, I removed the gauze and swabbed the socket with iodine. A tank of fresh seawater had been prepared for Panchito and when I gave the word he was dropped into it. He sank lazily to the bottom, gulping faintly. Soon the benzocaine's effects would wear off and the grouper would wake up in a temporary new home; that should make him really bloody-minded and finger-happy!

Panchito made a fine recovery and when, after a week, he was being returned to his right and proper tank where the benzocaine-dosed water had been replaced by fresh, unadulterated briny, he took the tip off the aquarium director's thumb in the process. Panchito rules, OK?

'Is cheeky boy, no? Is comico, yes?' I said to Robert when he told me over the phone.

We both laughed, but Panchito had the last laugh: my finger went septic.

8

I caught this morning morning's minion, king-
　　dom of daylight's dauphin, dapple-dawn-drawn Falcon, in
　　　his riding
　　Of the rolling level underneath him steady air, and
　　　striding
High there, how he rung upon the rein of a wimpling wing
In his ecstasy! then off, off forth on swing,
　　As a skate's heel sweeps smooth on a bow-bend: the hurl
　　　and gliding
　　Rebuffed the big wind. My heart in hiding
Stirred for a bird, – the achieve of, the mastery of the
　　thing!

Gerard Manley Hopkins' lines went through my mind as I watched
Kashmuk the peregrine tiercel stoop to the lure, falling like a black
stone out of the roseate dawn sky. The first breath of the khamsin,
the warm wind from the Empty Quarter, stroked my face. To my
right stretched the sun-bleached massif of the Jebel Hafit, still in
shadow. Somewhere up there among its myriad parched ravines
survived the Arabian tahr and maybe, just maybe, a leopard or two.
To my left lay a few acres of lush tropical garden with date palms
shading pepper, egg-plant and fruit bushes and a cluster of pale
green villas in the middle. Beyond the walls of the garden the desert
began, first a mile or so of flat, stony sand dotted with scrub and
the littered bones of camel, sheep and rat, and then, rising in
sensuous golden lines, the dunes, rank upon rank, that ran for five
hundred miles across Saudi Arabia. In Al Ain it was the best time of
the day for working. At first light Sundar, the Indian bailiff of
Sheikh Talib's palaces and estates, had collected me from my hotel

in the oasis town of Al Ain on the Abu Dhabi/Oman border and brought me to the garden where His Excellency maintained several hundred hunting hawks.

Al Ain Zoo contains a large collection of animals, some like Komodo dragons, colobus monkeys, Arabian oryx (including the last wild-caught animal in captivity), houbara bustard, bongo and kob being of unusual interest. Most zoo men dream of a zoo without visitors, but Al Ain comes close to it by being open only three days a week and with virtually free entrance it is not expected to make money; in that sense it is one of the few truly non-commercial zoos. It is a vast place, created by a fence enclosing a chunk of virgin desert, dunes and all, where it is possible to get lost and, when the sun is high, into serious trouble from the heat. In the arid countryside around the zoo there is an abundance of animal life to be seen by the observant: wild bull camels wandering alone looking for trouble the nomadic flocks of sheep that thrive on almost nothing, foxes, including the elusive Ruppel's fox, that come raiding at night, snakes and scorpions, eagles and jays and francolins and, somewhere out there it now seems certain, the great Arabian oryx still surviving in the most inhospitable desert area of the world.

This was the zoo at which Chris Furley, our assistant, was permanently based. Now he had gone on vacation through the Far East for four weeks and I was standing in for him. As well as the animals in the zoo, our services were called for to attend the mammals and birds kept as private collections by many sheikhs in the United Arab Emirates. The Arab of the Gulf has a special love of certain creatures: antelopes, deer and certain birds. *The* bird for the Arab is undoubtedly the falcon, saker or peregrine, with which he hunts and in which he takes as much pride as an English gentleman might in his string of thoroughbreds. His knowledge of the sport of hawking is at least as detailed as the equivalent passion of the football or cricket aficionado. His second-favourite bird is the houbara bustard. This creature, about the size of a partridge, is not very attractive to our eyes although the male does display a fine show of tail feathers when courting. It has great beauty however for the Arab, even though it is also the main quarry for his falconry.

The sheikhs go a-hunting with their falcons each year, now usually to Pakistan where houbara still exist in reasonable numbers. In Arabia they are less easy to find and a party of falconers out in the desert will be satisfied if the hawks take but one in a fortnight's hunting. But still on the one hand they hunt the houbara while on the other some sheikhs are going to great lengths to rear the species in captivity. In Dubai recently Sheikh Mohammed, Minister of Defence, took me by moonlight to see his precious collection of houbara, several hundred birds housed in pens on the desert edge. A suitable habitat has been carefully created inside the pens with special food for the birds, attendants and a guard to keep folk away. The houbara is considered to be a highly nervous bird that dies of heart attack if you so much as look at it (although I have found it possible to hospitalise specimens for regular medical treatment without trouble), and Sheikh Mohammed stressed the importance of privacy for his beloved houbara. 'Not even my local veterinarian is allowed to come within a hundred yards of these pens,' he told me.

But the right royal treatment is reserved for the falcons themselves. Each is worth up to £50,000 or even more, yet some owners may begin the hunting season with as many as a hundred and finish with a mere handful. The balance are lost or injured or die from disease. The falcons live in quarters far more commodious and pleasant than their human servants and the ruler of Abu Dhabi, Sheikh Zayed, built a hill specially on which to put airy houses where his gorgeous black Japanese peregrines could live in comfort, two to a room and perched on velvet-covered blocks driven into a fresh, fine-sand floor that is changed every day. The noble birds feast on pigeons, presented live but with their wings brutally broken to immobilise them, white rats and guinea pigs. They are adorned with jesses of calf-skin with silver swivels and keep cool in high summer by means of air-conditioning. Their hoods hanging on gold pegs on the walls of their rooms are made of finest leather tooled in gold, embroidered and cockaded with flamingo feathers.

Sheikh Talib, whose prize peregrine Kashmuk was, provided almost equally sumptuous accommodation for his falcons. There was no air-conditioning, but each bird had an individual palm-frond lattice hut that wouldn't have looked out of place in a Club Mediterranée watering-hole, and was attended to hand, beak and foot by a small army of Pakistani falconers who lived crammed together in a hovel that no peregrine would have been seen dead in. Kashmuk, sleek, proud, fierce Kashmuk, who would fly out of the sun like a dart from the Gods to take a gazelle even as it dashed into cover, Kashmuk who had led a trio of falcons that struck an ostrich while on a hunting-trip in Africa and who had 'bound' to as many as a score of houbara in a morning, Kashmuk who hunted duck by the light of the full moon – he, Kashmuk, had a chased gold water-bowl while the other falcons drank from silver. He was worth over £50,000 and in the early hours of this morning his Pakistani attendant, Ali, who earned £4 a week and all found, had reported to Sundar the bailiff that something wasn't quite right with Kashmuk. Dr Chris was away: better send for his boss, Dr Taylor.

While no expense is spared on most aspects of falcon care in Arabia, the approach to illness in the birds is still generally primitive. Ancient remedies, often relying on little more than magic, are widely employed and modern therapy and methods of disease prevention make slow headway. The use of a burning cigarette-end to cauterise the lesions of pox virus infection, rubbing sores with an amulet, barbaric surgery and worthless potions imported from India and Lebanon – these things are in common use. Prevention of disease spread from the often heavily infected pigeons used as food is almost impossible to organise. Nevertheless, Chris with Andrew's guidance had begun to introduce twentieth-century medicine into some of the sheikhs' collections with excellent results. Andrew, a keen bird man and interested in falconry since his school days at Winchester, was in his element among the literally thousands of birds of prey kept in Abu Dhabi.

As Ali the falconer brought Kashmuk towards us on a gloved fist, I asked Sundar what was worrying them.

'Kashmuk was frightened yesterday, Ali thinks by a bloody eagle,' he said. 'Just as he was striking a houbara, out from the hills

141

came the big bird. Ali says when its shadow fell on Kashmuk he was shocked and lost his prey.' The Indian spat in the dust.

Fond as the Arab is of birds of prey, his admiration extends only up to hawks and falcons. The bigger species he regards as pests and nuisances that disturb the game, sending them either into cover for long periods or panicking out into the desert where they collapse from heat exhaustion. Either way they're bad for hunting and he shoots or traps them at every opportunity. Foreigners frequently try to impress the sheikhs by presenting them with gifts of eagles. They are accepted politely, of course, but end up the next day at the zoo in Al Ain, where behind the scenes there is always a room or two full of such magnificent, often rare but unwanted presents.

I knew that eagles would put falcons off their stroke but Kashmuk didn't strike me as the sort of bird to be disturbed for long. 'How is it affecting him now?' I asked.

'Something to do with his breathing.'

Ali arrived and presented the peregrine on an outstretched arm. Kashmuk was a magnificent creature, steel-blue with a gleaming dark head and broad 'moustache' stripe. He surveyed me arrogantly with bright black eyes and mewed petulantly. Then I saw his breathing. It was far too fast. Kashmuk was panting.

'You say this is since the incident with the eagle yesterday?' I asked Ali.

'Yes, Doctor. He breathes now like this day and night.'

'Even in the cool times?'

'Even in the cool. I went to him during the night. He was the same.'

'Put the hood on him, please. I want to listen to his chest.'

Ali deftly slipped a leather hood over the falcon's eyes and used his teeth and the fingers of his free hand to tighten the retaining thongs. He kept Kashmuk on his glove while I gently felt the bird's body and applied the stethoscope diaphragm to its ribs.

'Now hold him in both hands while I look down his throat.' I opened the powerful beak and inspected the pink lining of the mouth, the pointed tongue and the glistening pharynx. No sign of croup or worms or the trichomonas parasite. I listened again to the breathing. There was a thickness to it, an occasional faint rasping. All things considered, I had a pretty shrewd idea what was the matter with Kashmuk and the outlook couldn't have been grimmer. Down in the peregrine's lungs a mould looking exactly like the stuff that develops harmlessly on stale bread or the surface of a pot of jam was growing. Kashmuk was in the early stages of the deadly infection caused by aspergillus fungus.

I'd seen a lot of aspergillus in my zoo work. It can occur in young turkeys, other species of birds and occasionally mammals including man, and it is very common among birds of prey, but most of all you will find it wreaking havoc among my favourite sort of bird, the penguins. Lower the resistance, be it ever so subtly, of a penguin, perhaps just by moving it from A to B or changing its diet – or even, I sometimes think, by just looking at it – and the fungus infection is likely to break out. Penguins do have other diseases like malaria and foot problems but in 99.9% of cases if a penguin falls ill you can bet it's aspergillus. Like other fungus infections inside the body it is very difficult to treat – antibiotics probably make it worse – and at the time of Kashmuk's attack his chances of recovery could be regarded as zero.

'What do you think, Doctor?' asked Sundar. 'Upset by the eagle?'

'No,' I replied, 'Kashmuk has got radad.' I used the Arabic word for the disease, literally translatable as 'the mushroom that grows in the lungs'.

Both men looked stunned. 'Radad, Doctor? Radad?' exclaimed Sundar. 'But this is Kashmuk! If he dies His Excellency will . . . will . . . I don't know. But maybe you should get your bags packed ready!'

'I can't help it getting radad. It's a very serious infection. Sheikh Talib must accept that.'

Sundar shrugged and smiled apologetically. A genial, quick-witted man who spoke half a dozen languages fluently and administered his master's estates with consummate skill, he understood intimately both the Arab and the European mind. 'He can accept disease and death, Doctor. To the Muslim that is the will of Allah, fate, kismet. But having called you in, you the specialist in animal diseases not from Lahore or Bombay or Damascus but from London, things are changed. Now it's no longer in the hands of Allah alone. You have, how shall I say, interfered with the outcome of things. Failure on your part he could not accept.'

'That,' I retorted grimly, 'is an Islamic each-way bet. Suppose I hadn't been here?'

'We would do our best with the old ways, forcing the bird to take the urine of a young camel mulled with a hot poker.'

'And when Kashmuk had then gone ahead and died, would he have accepted what you'd done?'

'Yes. But from you in the West, although you are secretly and profoundly looked down upon by the Bedou, much is expected of your science. They pay well and expect success.'

'From the infidels.'

'From the infidels, Doctor.' Sundar patted me on the shoulder and motioned Ali to take the falcon back to its room. 'Come, Doctor. Let us have some suleimani tea while you tell me what we must do.'

While I sat with Sundar in his office at the edge of the garden, drinking the sweet red tea and watching the hoopoes flit across the palms, I pondered over the problem of Kashmuk. Soon his breathing would become laboured. His appetite would go. After a few days, maybe a week, his lungs would be swamped by the green and white mould and would pack up. A human afflicted by such a complaint could be given fungus-killing drugs such as miconazole, but they had to be dripped in slowly and precisely over several hours by way of an intravenous transfusion and there was no chance of doing that with a falcon. Inhalations had been tried on penguins – making them breathe in drug-laden vapours – but hadn't proved very successful. Medicines in the food or water were no better. Of the few anti-fungal preparations available, most weren't absorbed from the bowels of a bird and the rest didn't kill the aspergillus fungus. Perhaps if I rigged up some sort of oxygen tent in Kashmuk's room it would help. At least it would give me a breathing-space to consider the matter back at my hotel and have a natter with Andrew on the telephone.

144

I told Sundar to obtain oxygen and an oxygen tent. When one of His Excellency's falcons is ill it takes precedence over everything and everybody except the Sheikh and his family. Al Ain has several well-equipped hospitals, some of them for the exclusive use of Emirate nationals and built with special self-contained wings and separate operating theatres for dignitaries. If I broke my neck outside one of these places, as a foreigner I wouldn't get inside, but a call from the Sheikh's office commanding a complete oxygen unit to be delivered to the falcon houses in the garden brought one within the hour – under police escort with sirens wailing and lights flashing. Kashmuk certainly had pull!

Once back at my hotel I telephoned Andrew. It was four o'clock in the morning in England when I woke him to discuss the falcon.

'There's just been a report published in a German journal,' he said sleepily after hearing me out. 'Something about using one of these human intravenous drugs on penguins with aspergillus but given by ordinary intramuscular injection. As far as I can tell they had excellent results although they're reporting on only five or six cases. You'll need to get Hanne to translate the piece. There isn't much of it.'

'Great. Do me a favour, ring Hanne now and get her started. Then ask her to ring me with the translation. Best of luck when she finds you waking her up at this hour!'

Half an hour later Hanne telephoned. She was not amused, but she'd quickly translated the words that Andrew had awkwardly read out to her. It was true: a vet in Germany seemed to have saved a handful of infected penguins with a series of miconazole injections.

I went back to Sheikh Talib's garden to talk to Sundar. 'I might be able to do something with a new injection,' I told him.

Sundar looked at me pensively and raised his eyebrows. 'Injection, you say, Doctor? Ah well, I'm not sure what His Excellency will feel about that.'

'What do you mean? I thought my job was to come up with the miracle cure.'

He laughed. 'It is. It is. But an injection, that's the problem. We'll need his permission for that.'

'To inject?'

'I'm afraid so. He loves Kashmuk very dearly, you know. Injections mean going to have an audience with His Excellency.'

We'd had similar difficulties before. The Doctor from England must do everything necessary to cure the beast but not this or that or that and certainly not *that*. Pills and potions and lotions and liniments were acceptable forms of medicine; injections, surgery, adjustments of diet were not. One sheikh had a large herd of Arabian oryx that he kept in a garden. An epidemic of foot-and-mouth disease had struck them and losses had been high. While we wrestled with controlling the virus as best we could, the sheikh blamed the pestilence on poisons in the fresh lucerne which formed the bulk of the animals' diet. Part of our proposed treatment was to dart the oryx with supportive drugs and also to boost the level of nutrition by adding concentrate pellets to the food. Permission was not given. We must 'get the animals right' without darts or injections or new-fangled food pellets and the lucerne was to be stopped at once. This left the animals with nothing to eat but plain barley. In the event we took a risk and slipped the oryx bales of lucerne in the evenings when we were sure the sheikh was not due to pay a visit. We did not dare dart them; informers would have blown the whistle on us within minutes, for Arabia has eyes everywhere.

On another occasion we were rendered even more impotent when a virus epidemic decimated a vast paddock-full of gazelles. The dart-rifle was the only way to tackle the problem, but the command for us to treat the animals immediately was coupled to another which said that there must be no darting. We sprayed antiseptic over hundreds of square yards of sand for days on end, said our prayers and left it at that. As is the way with Mother Nature, when she had wiped out eighty per cent of the gazelle herd she called it a day, the deaths ceased and for our 'success' in treating the holocaust Chris was presented with a gold watch!

And now it looked as if I might face a similar problem with Kashmuk. I was worried enough about using an untried drug on a falcon, let alone such a stupendously valuable one, without having

146

to beg for permission to use it! Suppose it was toxic for peregrines. Penguins in Germany are a whole lot different from falcons in Arabia. Why, oh why, hadn't I got faith in mulled camel urine? 'Arrange me an audience as soon as you can, please,' I said. 'Meanwhile I'll try to find the drug in Abu Dhabi.'

It turned out that none of the pharmacies, hospitals or veterinary clinics in the whole of Abu Dhabi had the intravenous miconazole solution. I phoned Andrew to get some put on the next plane from Heathrow. Kashmuk wasn't breathing any worse under his transparent oxygen tent, but then again there wasn't much improvement. He looked like lasting at least until I could start the series of injections – if I got permission from his master.

Later in the day Sundar called at the little veterinary laboratory which is our centre of operations in Al Ain Zoo. 'His Excellency will speak to you at his majlis at seven o'clock tonight. He's just had a tooth pulled and is not in a very good mood. I'll pick you up at a little before seven.'

Just my luck, I thought. Audiences with Arab sheikhs are tricky and imprecise enough without dentists doing their worst. It's just the excuse he'll need for not turning up, I mused glumly. Then tomorrow there'll be something else: a summons from Sheikh Zayed for him to meet some visiting head of state from overseas or he'll disappear for a few days to one of his palaces on the coast and I'll have to kick my heels waiting for permission to unsheath my trusty hypodermic and all the time Kashmuk is getting worse and my head is nearing the chopping block. Sheikh-hunting, predicting where they'll be at what time and for how long, has much in common with playing roulette.

Sheikh Talib held his majlis, or audience, in one of his smaller palaces near the town centre of Al Ain. After taking off our shoes we entered a large, richly carpeted room containing a photograph of the Ruler and a television set as its only furniture. The set was switched on and the 'Muppet Show' blared out at full volume. Men in dish-dashes sat or sprawled round the walls. At the far end, in cream-coloured robes, squatted His Excellency. A small round man with a reddish beard and eyebrows, he looked grumpy and kept rubbing his cheek. Everyone stood as we walked in and, beginning with the Sheikh, did the rounds of shaking hands and exchanging the traditional 'salaam' greeting. Sheikh Talib did not speak English but motioned for me to sit next to him with Sundar on my other side. A servant dispensed cups of bitter Arab coffee and then, battling against the din of the Muppets, we did the Arab equivalent of talking about the weather, exchanging pleasantries with one of His Excellency's companions or another, but never with the Sheikh himself, about how London was getting on, was it true that Islam was sweeping through England (Arabs are never reticent about speaking of religion in general conversation), and did it feel strange having a woman as Prime Minister. From time to time there were long periods when nobody spoke and the floor was left to the Muppets. Once or twice I caught the Sheikh scrutinising me, doubtfully I felt, but he said nothing. At last, when I was almost awash with coffee, Sheikh Talib clicked his fingers and sent a servant away for something. The man came back carrying some boxes of fruit. He set the boxes down at the Sheikh's feet and bowed his way out. His Excellency stuck his hand into one box and pulled out a fistful of small medlars. These he proceeded to roll across the somewhat grubby carpet, some for each of the assembled company. He grunted towards me in Arabic. 'His Excellency says ''Eat'','' translated Sundar. I picked up the first of the medlars, fluffy with bits of carpet dust and God knows what else, grinned at our host and began to eat. When I'd finished the last of my medlars the Sheikh began to roll more towards me and grunted again. '''Eat,'' His Excellency says,' repeated Sundar. 'Does the English Doctor not like the fruit from his farm?'

'Oh yes, yes,' I said, stuffing another medlar down. 'First-class fruit, very tasty. Please tell His Excellency so.'

To my horror, when the medlars were finished, Sheikh Talib started on another box, this time of ripe cherries sticky with juice where their skins were splitting. They gathered more debris as they were rolled around the floor but I manfully ate my share. Dear Lord, let me survive gastro-enteritis long enough at least to start Kashmuk's treatment after all this, I prayed.

148

The cherries lasted longer than the medlars and then came the pièce de resistance. The Sheikh dug into a third box to extract what looked like handfuls of sticky worms, rolled them accurately in my direction and said to me, 'Toot, toot.'

'Toot,' said Sundar. 'Toot.'

I looked at him and then back at the 'worms'. They were in fact a long, gooey sort of fruit that I'd never seen before in my life.

'Toot, toot,' said the Sheikh again and prodded his cheek irritably.

Gone mad, I thought. 'Toot,' I said tentatively. 'What does that mean, Sundar?'

'That is what it is. There is no English translation as far as I know. This fruit is called "toot" in Arabic. Try it.'

The toot really did resemble earthworms and their gooey texture had done an even tidier job of cleaning the shag pile. 'Toot, toot,' I said, trying to grin again and popping one in my mouth. It tasted rather like an anaemic raspberry.

'His Excellency says you should eat, Doctor. You'll not find toot as good as his back in England, he says. Eat!'

After another half-hour of 'tooting' His Excellency suddenly directed a question at Sundar. The Indian replied at length in rapid Arabic. Then, turning to me he said, 'Sheikh Talib wants to know what you are doing here instead of Dr Chris.'

'I have come because Dr Chris is on vacation,' I replied, rather taken aback.

'His Excellency says he knows Dr Chris and can't understand why he's not here if Kashmuk is sick.'

'Dr Chris, my assistant, went on vacation before Kashmuk became ill, please tell His Excellency. He is now somewhere in Singapore. That is why he isn't here.'

Sundar translated and waited for Sheikh Talib's next sally. 'His Excellency likes Dr Chris.'

'So do I.'

'He hasn't met you before.'

'Neither have I met His Excellency before.' This was becoming ridiculous. 'Make it quite clear, Sundar, that Dr Chris works for me. What Dr Chris would do, I will do also.'

There was a couple of minutes pause and then: 'His Excellency can't understand why Dr Chris isn't here. He knows Dr Chris.'

Patience, boy, I told myself. Keep your cool. Don't lose face. Then I said, 'Please tell His Excellency that I am the Professor of Peregrine Falcons from the University of Wigan in England. There is nothing I don't know or haven't done concerning falcons, or anything else for that matter. I can revive oven-ready chickens, unblock stuffed-up parson's noses and make a damned good soufflé out of a curate's egg. If I carry on like this I might one day be fit to carry the bag of my good friend, Dr Chris. In the meanwhile I would like to try treating Kashmuk!'

Sundar listened intently to my monologue and then without comment addressed the Sheikh again. He had to speak loudly because of Miss Piggy. I have no idea what Sundar said in Arabic but His Excellency's sour expression did not alter in the slightest as he listened. Then he made a brief remark.

'His Excellency wishes to know what you propose to do about poor Kashmuk.'

'Tell him that, as he knows, radad is very, very serious. I wish to try a new treatment to cure the falcon. I can do my best, that is all.'

Sundar conferred again with the Sheikh. 'His Excellency says can the new treatment be given in the food?'

'No.'

More conferring. The Muppets' singing continued to thunder round the room. 'His Excellency would prefer the treatment to be given in the food.'

'It can't. It must be by injection.' I made a syringe-injecting gesture with one hand. Sheikh Talib was looking distinctly grumpier and was cupping one side of his face in a hand.

'His Excellency doesn't like injections.'

'Neither do I, but tell him it is the only way.'

Sundar chattered away again and the Sheikh grunted something. 'His Excellency says the Pakistani vets have some drops that they put in the birds' water.'

150

'I know. It's rubbish for radad.' How long must this crazy bargaining go on, I wondered, as they talked again and Kermit the frog ranted away behind them.

'Will the injection work, His Excellency asks.'

'Insh' Allah,' I replied. 'If God wills.'

Suddenly Sheikh Talib slapped his offending cheek and gave a soft groan. He nodded once, said a few more words to Sundar and got to his feet.

'You can do it. He says you can inject Kashmuk,' exclaimed Sundar quickly, his face lighting up as we too stood. 'His Excellency must go now. His jaw is giving him pain.'

Hands were shaken and blessings intoned once again and the men began to melt away. The audience was over. With the help of the demoralising effects of a rough time in the dentist's chair, I'd been given the go-ahead to have a real crack at the sick peregrine. But what if the new miconazole treatment turned out to be a disaster? I tried not to think about that as I went back to the zoo. My assistant had left me strict instructions while he was away to water all his house-plants regularly. After doing the watering and feeding the jaguar cub he was rearing I would raid his refrigerator for an Amstel or two before settling down to plan a treatment regime for Kashmuk, to be begun as soon as the miracle drug arrived from England.

'Just one thing, Doctor,' said Sundar as he dropped me off. 'His Excellency said you can give the injection, but that it must work. Kashmuk hunts in Pakistan next month.'

'Great!' I muttered, as his car disappeared into the darkness and the gibbons in their cage outside the laboratory hooted and chirruped with mirth. I turned into the laboratory to check with Andrew by telephone that the miconazole had been safely delivered to Heathrow.

'Oh, and Liliana's rung from Madrid,' my partner told me when he had confirmed that the drug should be on its way. 'Chang-Chang the panda is passing occasional lumps of mucus in his droppings. It seems to be associated with periods of lassitude and loss of appetite but it always clears up spontaneously after no more than twenty-four hours.'

It seemed that troubles never came singly. 'Ring her back and ask her to send some samples of the mucus by air and kept as fresh as possible packed in ice inside a thermos flask,' I told Andrew. 'Then get them straight to the laboratory for analysis.'

Next day Kashmuk's respiration on his block inside the oxygen tent was more laboured. He turned down every sort of food offered to him by Ali. I drove the ninety miles across the desert to the airport in Dubai, only to find that the parcel of miconazole injection had somehow stayed on the ground at Heathrow when the Gulf Air flight departed. Seething, I stayed overnight in the city to await the next plane. Twelve hours and a small bribe to a customs official later, I had my precious injections. I returned post haste to Al Ain and went straight to see Kashmuk.

'He is worse, Doctor,' moaned Ali the falconer. 'Listen to the hoarseness now in his breath. O, may a thousand djinns carry fire-brands up the fundament of that accursed eagle and burn out its liver!'

'Ali, Kashmuk is not sick because of the eagle's shadow. It is a germ, a microbe.'

'So you say, Doctor, but I have been a falconer since I was a lad and my father before me and my grandfather before him. He was falconer to the Viceroy of India. What you call a germ, Doctor, we know to be the shadow.'

'OK. Let's see how the injection works on the shadow then. Please hood him and hold him with both hands.'

When the peregrine was secured I filled my tiny syringe with the miconazole liquid, fitted my finest needle and, keeping my fingers out of reach of the powerful talons, injected into the breast muscle of the bird.

On each of the nine following mornings I was up early with Omar Khayyam as the 'hunter of the East' caught the Sultan's, or at least Sheikh Talib's, turret in a noose of light. While the muezzins were calling the faithful to work and prayer, I set out for the garden to give Kashmuk his daily injection. By the third injection I fancied I could detect some easing of the bird's breathing although he still lacked all appetite and had to be carefully force-fed with steak dipped in beaten egg. Then to my delight, halfway through the course the harsh rattling inside his lungs faded distinctly. On the sixth day he started eating voluntarily. The miconazole was undoubtedly destroying the disease-producing fungus.

'See how the new drug works a miracle!' I said to Ali.

'He is forgetting the eagle's shadow,' the Pakistani replied, 'and yes, he is improving, Doctor.'

I was highly excited by the apparent results of the new therapy. Radad, aspergillosis in falcons, looked like being combatable for the first time since falconry began to be practised in China around 2000 BC. On the day of the final injection I talked to Andrew on the telephone and told him how Kashmuk, now out of the oxygen tent, was back to normal, breathing easily and eating voraciously.

'This is certainly going to revolutionise penguin and falcon work,' said my partner, 'but there's one thing you should know. Just after you began Kashmuk's treatment, I used the injection on a rock-hopper penguin with terrible fungus lungs. It was amazingly better after the third shot, but unfortunately then a fox got it. I did the p-m this morning. Sure enough the aspergillus was beating a hasty retreat but where the drug had been injected into the breast muscles I found quite a bit of muscle damage.'

The implications of Andrew's remark didn't hit me at first. True, the injection was intended for intravenous use in humans; drugs in that form sometimes are irritant, a property unnoticeable and unimportant in the bloodstream but producing reaction and occasionally pain when injected under the skin or into muscle.

'Did the penguin show any sign of pain when injected?' I asked. 'Kashmuk didn't seem to notice them at all.'

'No, not a bit. But there are some nasty white lines in the breast muscle.'

'I suppose it can't be helped,' I said. 'A bit of soreness is better than dying choking, and the muscle will quickly scar over.'

Then I felt a little icicle beginning to form in the pit of my stomach. Breast muscle — the commonest, safest, easiest muscle to use for injecting any species of bird — breast muscle, the tasty white meat that everyone fancies slices off when the Christmas turkey is brought in: breast muscle powers the wings. Penguins, or Christmas turkeys, have breast muscles galore but don't, can't fly. Penguins in zoos don't have to swim strongly underwater. Some reaction, even a bit of muscle damage and scarring in their bosoms, wouldn't matter one iota. But falcons, especially the once mighty Kashmuk, are nothing if they are not power fliers. They are eyes and breast muscles in a supremely orchestrated combination. Earlier estimates of the speed of a peregrine's stoop (up to 250 mph) are now discounted and analysis of ciné film has shown that the bird levels and slows slightly before striking at about 40 mph. But its thrilling plunges from the heavens are the most dramatic of all the hawks and everything depends on the correct functioning of the breast muscles.

'Have you tried Kashmuk flying again?' Andrew asked.

'No, not yet.' I felt rather numb. 'I must see what he can do tomorrow.'

'Well, here's something else for you. I've had the lab report on the stool analysis from Chang-Chang. There were no parasites or germs, nothing significant. The mucus was just mucus – clear, structureless jelly. I've been on the phone to the vets at the National Zoo in Washington and they've seen the same thing occasionally, but they don't know the reason for it.'

I pondered. 'Let's do nothing for the moment. Maybe normal pandas do pass mucus once in a while. But I don't like the sound of those associated periods of lethargy and loss of appetite.'

Andrew rang off and I was contemplating my fate if it transpired that, in curing Kashmuk's lungs, I had rendered him permanently earth-bound, when Sundar telephoned. 'His Excellency will come to the garden to see Kashmuk's progress in the cool of the evening tomorrow. It would be best if you were there.'

'I'll be there,' I replied and thought, Please God make falcons out of tougher material than penguins.

The fateful day dawned and started badly; the omens concerning Sheikh Talib were grim, to say the least, for shortly after the zoo gates opened a Cadillac rolled into the grounds and a cluster of small Arab children spilled out, followed by two sinister-looking Bedou men carrying sub-machine guns. This was Al Ain Zoo's equivalent of harassed nuns shepherding a convent-school biology class round Regent's Park or Chester: the children of a sheikh out for a day at the zoo in the care of bodyguards. I had seen such parties many times. Screeching and shouting, the children and their minders disappeared from my view up the walk towards the giraffe house.

Some time later, as I sat in the laboratory looking at a blood smear under the microscope, Peter, one of the English curators, burst through the door. 'Bloody hell,' he bellowed. 'I just do not believe it. That beats all!' He flung himself down onto a chair, his face red with anger, and glared at me.

I'd known Peter since we'd worked together at several zoos in the North of England. An uncompromising and dedicated animal man, he did not suffer fools gladly. I'd seen him duff up some oaf of a keeper at Flamingo Park who had, through negligence, allowed two of Peter's beloved bigs cats to injure themselves in a fight. But I'd never seen him as irate as this. 'What's up?' I asked.

For a minute he could barely control himself enough to get the words out. Then he spluttered, 'The ostrich. The ostrich. Those bloody kids are stoning the ostrich eggs.'

Each year the ostriches at Al Ain laid eggs and hatched them, although we were having trouble rearing the youngsters which tended to outgrow their strength and to develop bone disease. The eggs were laid in a shallow depression scooped out of the sandy paddock and guarded by the mother and the exceedingly pugnacious red-neck father. This year, however, the clutch of huge eggs lay within stone-throwing distance of the public.

I stood up to make for the door. 'Didn't you stop them?' I asked.

'Of course I did. At least I tried to.' Peter waved me away from the door. 'It's no use you going. The bodyguards won't let you interfere.'

'What do you mean?'

'Those kids are Sheikh Talib's brood. They thought it wonderful sport to chuck stones at the eggs. Broke one before my eyes. I dashed up yelling and then it happened.'

'What happened?'

'As soon as I approached one of the kids who was organising the throwing to give him an earful, one of the guards unslung his gun and stuck it right here.' He pointed at his stomach. 'Stuck it in my belly and said shove off, let them have their fun.'

Peter's Arabic is not bad. He had got the message: if a sheikh's favourites want to break a few eggs, so what's the hassle? Anyway, it's the custom of Arab bodyguards to carry weapons loaded with live ammunition and with one round up the spout, and the muzzle of the Sterling Mark 4 seemed a comfortable fit in Peter's navel.

'You think he'd have pulled the trigger if you'd persisted and gone ahead and restrained the little monster?'

'Talib's men have a bad reputation. ''Accidents'' with loaded guns happen all the time. Talib is a hard case, David.'

When the Cadillac eventually purred out of the zoo we went to count the cost. Three eggs were smashed and one cracked. While Peter held the red-neck at bay with a broom, I made emergency repairs, filling the crack with plaster of Paris and coating it with nail varnish. Such tribulations occur in all zoos. They are just writ uncommonly large in the Middle East.

Later in the day I went as usual with Sundar to inspect Kashmuk. He looked in the pink. Surely that firm chest would operate his wings satisfactorily. 'Bring him outside,' I told Ali. 'I want you to fly Kashmuk to a lure. Just a short distance to see whether he's feeling himself.'

Ali prepared a dead pigeon on the end of a length of cord as a lure and then brought the peregrine out into the fierce sunshine. He cast out the lure a distance of perhaps ten yards and then released the falcon. Kashmuk spread his wings, flapped them feebly and launched himself – only to land, looking rather surprised with himself, halfway between Ali and the lure. It was a heavy landing.

The falconer clicked his teeth and muttered something under his breath in Urdu.

'Er . . . he's a bit convalescent, naturally,' I said with what I hoped was a ring of confidence. 'I'll give him a shot of tonic, I think.' I took some anti-inflammatory steroid injection out of my bag.

'Do you think he'll be OK by tonight when His Excellency inspects him?' Sundar sounded very doubtful.

'Well, we'll see,' I replied, filling the syringe.

'But we must hunt in Pakistan in two weeks,' said Ali gloomily. He spat a blood-red pool of betel nut onto the ground a millimetre in front of my shoe.

My heart wasn't in my work when I returned to the zoo. I took Chris's Suzuki jeep and drove out into the desert, stripped off and lay prone on the sand. The breeze whistled gently. There was no other sound. I watched a column of tiny ants, the ones that can really sting, go to and fro a foot from my nose. They were putting the finishing touches to a shining white camel skull that projected from the sand close by. 'If Kashmuk is ruined,' I said out loud to the gleaming skull, 'my future in Arabia might be as bright as yours, my friend.'

When the sun was low and the day began to cool, Sundar collected me in his car and we drove to meet Sheikh Talib at the garden. The sky had turned from blue to a wash of contrasting water-colours that merged with one another dramatically. Deep purple swirled into yellow and that into smoky brown and lakes of pearl.

'Looks very pretty,' I said.

'Looks like bad weather,' replied Sundar. 'See the dust-devils coming.'

I looked across the flat near-desert. Whirling clouds of dust, no bigger than the size of a man, were dancing across the land.

'The old folk really believe they are djinns on the warpath,' Sundar told me.

As we turned into the garden the date palms were nodding anxiously before the rising wind. The horizon towards the hazy sun was fuzzy and dark. We drove straight to the villas in the centre of the garden. I could tell by the collection of limousines drawn up that His Excellency had arrived. We found him sitting on a terrace sipping sherbet. He was surrounded by men, some of whom were carrying hawks on their gloved wrists. Others had drawn to one end of the terrace and were unhurriedly performing their evening prayers, kneeling on small oblongs of carpet. After the formalities of greeting, Sheikh Talib got straight down to business. He seemed to be in a less saturnine mood and there was no sign of trouble with his mouth, although I imagined he scowled at me from time to time. 'Where is Dr Chris? Why is he not here?' he opened up through Sundar.

Not that again! I counted to ten. 'Dr Chris is still away in the Far East. He can't be contacted but is coming soon. I'm still here.'

The Sheikh slurped his sherbet noisily as he reflected for a few moments. 'Have you injected Kashmuk?'

'Yes. The drug seems to have cured the radad.'

'And Kashmuk is himself again?'

'Yes, well, no. Such a serious illness needs a period to regain strength.'

'Tell Ali Prathan to bring Kashmuk. We will see him fly.' His Excellency snapped out the order and a servant scuttled out.

The sun was now a bloody stain on the blurred horizon. The noise of the wind rose in the bushes and trees of the garden. I saw the men at the edge of the terrace squint their eyes and became aware of stinging particles of sand and dust in the air. 'Sand-storm,' whispered Sundar to me as we watched Ali come trotting through the trees with the falcon, his garments fluttering wildly. Kashmuk was hooded and calmly sat staring blindly into the wind that ruffled his breast plumage. As the falconer reached the steps leading up to the terrace the sky darkened as if smoke had been instantaneously released all around us. A cloud of buzzing sand swept across the garden and into the terrace. The grit prickled my eyes, nose, mouth and ears and stung my scalp. Everything became indistinct and monochromatic brown. 'Into the villa,' ordered Sundar, grabbing my arm. His Excellency was already inside. Ali and Kashmuk were ushered in close behind him.

'We cannot fly Kashmuk in here,' said the Sheikh when we were all resettled around the walls of a tapestried but otherwise empty room. I listened with satisfaction to the howling outside and watched the hurrying fog outside the window continue unabated. 'You say, Doctor, that all is well. He looks well. Does he eat well?'

'Most satisfactorily.'

'Get a pigeon.'

A man went out and returned shortly covered in dust and carrying a live pigeon. Deftly the man dislocated its wings, locked them behind its back and threw it on the floor.

'Release Kashmuk.'

The peregrine did his stuff with terrible efficiency.

'Unfortunately I must leave tonight for Abu Dhabi. I am sorry I cannot see Kashmuk fly.' The Sheikh scowled at me quite plainly. 'Now your injections are finished, do you think Kashmuk will hunt well in two weeks?'

'I trust so, Your Excellency.'

Saved by a sand-storm – it raged for another three hours – I returned to my hotel in high spirits and with sand in every crevice of my body. Worrying about Kashmuk and his demonstration had put me off my food; now I ordered a couple of hammour fish steaks, a bowl of tahina and a bottle of Pinot Grigio. I had two weeks' reprieve, courtesy of the desert wind, to sort out Kashmuk.

The peregrine's muscles, inflamed by the miconazole injection, must have caused him soreness when he tried to fly, but gradually as the days passed the reaction died down. He continued to eat strongly and I instructed Ali to give him a graded programme of exercise. Drops of anti-inflammatory medicine in his water helped as well. He began to fly more surely to the lure and at last, one bright morning when all was still and the full moon still hung in the sky over the mountains as the sun turned their jagged ramparts from purple into pink, Sundar, Ali and I took the peregrine out into the desert. The proud tiercel was unhooded, the lure was cast far out and with a triumphant cry from the falconer Kashmuk rose into the warming air and made for the paling moon. His long wings winnowed the air as he climbed. Then, reaching some invisible peak, he rolled elegantly to one side and came scything down through the crystal air. He struck the lure perfectly, stood proudly for a second, his feathers gilded by the sun, and then began to tear at the pigeon meat.

'The shadow has gone, Ali,' I said.

'Aye, the shadow has gone, Doctor. Kashmuk will go hunting in Pakistan.' The falconer walked towards his bird, calling softly.

Kashmuk did go hunting and hunted well, and while he was away my assistant came back from leave and I returned to England.

A few weeks later Chris phoned to say he'd had an audience with Sheikh Talib. 'He's very pleased with Kashmuk,' he told me. 'Ever so pleased to see me, too. I got the impression he wasn't all that keen on you, though. And guess what – he's giving me a present of a Range Rover. Not a bad old bugger, eh?'

9

The warden in charge of the big cats at Windsor Safari Park took another look through his binoculars and gasped loud enough to cause his assistant, who was keeping his eyes firmly fixed on a tiger that was sneaking slowly towards the electrically operated gate, to turn his head.

'What the devil?' muttered the warden. 'The cheetahs are dancing about!' He handed over the glasses and pointed to the distant cheetah reserve. 'Have a quick look and then we'll drive over. Rummest thing I ever saw. Dancing cheetahs!'

The two men climbed into the zebra-painted Land Rover and drove across the grassy parkland, avoiding the snake of visitors' cars making their way through the Berkshire bit of darkest Africa on a late Sunday afternoon in July. The cheetahs were in their favourite corner of the reserve, a quiet shaded area where Gary Smart and I had ordered the grass and weeds to be allowed to grow unchecked some years before in order to create some privacy for the mating of these shy and easily distracted cats. (It seemed to have worked; we had begun to breed cheetahs and had even had one female who presented a litter of six cubs.) When they drew close to the animals, the two wardens found their initial impressions apparently confirmed; it did look like dancing. The leggy, spotted cats that we'd imported from south-west Africa were milling about in the most extraordinary way. It looked like some sort of feline hoe-down, everyone moving in circles or going to and fro, claws lifted abnormally high in a high-stepping gait and rumps and tails swaying to some exotic rhythm outside the range of human ears. Not only that but like African ritual dancers in a trance, they seemed unaware of the Land Rover's arrival; expressions were fixed, eyes stared into infinity and soft mewings came from half-opened mouths.

'Is it some sort of mating display like birds do?' The assistant wasn't experienced in the ways of big cats, but his boss wasn't listening. He was already calling up Francis Rendell, the park's curator, on his walkie-talkie.

'Cheetahs all haywire,' he was saying. 'Gone bonkers or food-poisoned or something. Better get the vet in fast.'

When he looked back to the weird ballet he saw that two of the animals had collapsed and were lying apparently unconscious. A third was finishing its pas de quatre with a downward-spiralling collapse onto its haunches to sit as immobile as a Staffordshire china dog. That left six carrying on with the choreography. The warden looked round; there were more cheetahs somewhere. He caught sight of them lying on their sides in a patch of sunlight thirty yards away. They looked as cool and poised as ever. He walked towards them and when he got as close as they were prepared to allow they stood up, stared at him and stamped their fore-feet in warning before turning and loping fluidly away. No dancing or unconsciousness there. The warden hurried back to the unconscious cheetahs, which looked to be flat out. He pulled at the tongue of one that was threatening to choke and cursed as the furry dancers reeled round him.

I had just finished talking to Liliana in Madrid about another attack of Chang-Chang's listlessness – again it was accompanied by mucus in the droppings but again we had decided on balance not to interfere – when Francis rang. 'Can you come over right away? Looks like bad food-poisoning.' I'd worked with Francis, one of the most widely experienced of young British zoo curators and a first-class marine mammal man, for many years by then. An imperturbable character who had coped, cool as a cucumber, with innumerable alarums in the zoo world, he sounded unusually hot and bothered. Something very serious must be up.

'I'm on my way. Meanwhile brew up some very strong black coffee – about half a gallon,' I said after he'd briefly described the symptoms. 'I'll explain when I get there.'

162

The move to Lightwater had been advantageous in more ways than one. Now I was only twenty minutes from the Windsor park. It made more sense for me to be in the South and leave Andrew to handle the North, even though it meant that I rarely visited dear old Belle Vue. In the past I'd sometimes driven twice in one day from Rochdale to London or Windsor. The long motorway run didn't trouble me, but I had collected speeding fines with monotonous regularity, stiff necks from cat-napping in lay-bys and service stations and indigestion from hurried meals-on-wheels. With the radio-telephone in my car I'd been able to handle most distant emergencies well enough, but there's no substitute for getting to a case as fast as possible. With the best will in the world, and a police escort on occasion, it is still impossible to cover the 200-odd miles between Lancashire and London in less than two and a half hours – long enough by far for many urgent cases to pass beyond the point of no return. I'd been lucky over the years, but now our dispositions were more logical and secure. Francis's cheetahs illustrated the point perfectly.

From the telephone description I suspected poisoning, not from food but from something more sinister – malicious doping. It is not infrequent, and I see one or two cases per year in zoo carnivores. Zoos attract cranks and nutters among their visitors and they also regularly produce disgruntled staff, individuals with chips on their shoulders who become obsessed with the animals in their care, spend long hours alone communing with bird or beast, and gradually lose their sense of perspective. Grudges may be incubated against the head keeper or director who are seen as unsympathetic or downright cruel in, say, deciding to sell a particular favourite creature or refusing to supply some item of diet that is not strictly necessary but which a keeper would like to please his charges with. There are a thousand and one areas where seeds of resentment may grow in every zoo. Zoo staff are generally poorly paid in comparison to workers in other industries; many are dedicated idealists who do not share the aims and attitudes of management towards captive animals. Management often communicates poorly or not at all with the people who are actually in charge, day in and day out, of stock worth perhaps millions of pounds. The man who has to muck out the monkeys is rarely if ever consulted when the architects roll up in their limousines to sketch out the new monkey house, so it doesn't surprise you to learn that the said house, when erected in arty-crafty stainless steel and given a champagne opening by Sir Solly Zuckerman or whoever, like as not hasn't got anywhere for the monkey-man to dump his muck.

Strangely, animal staff who are dismissed for some reason and, even more strangely, animal staff who are still in employment at the zoo, may occasionally go bad and strike back for real or imagined grievances not against the directorate but against the inmates themselves: the animals. Paradoxically, the animal man rounds on his animals. I see much of this phenomenon. Giraffes deliberately terrorised at night in the darkness of their houses – four dead of shock by first light. Arson that killed a house full of parrots and nearly cost the lives of zebra and bison. Stabbings and shootings of monkeys and birds. No, I'm not referring to incidents that might have been the work of the public, of vandals breaking in after hours: these are known cases where zoo staff have lost their grip on reason. Where the culprits have tried to explain their motives, not once have I heard anything about an inexplicable hatred of the animals having arisen in their minds. The explanations, sometimes tortuous, sometimes startlingly lucid, have always outlined humans or human systems as the foe. 'Anyone who works with animals in whatever capacity must be at least a bit dotty,' says a zoo director friend. He may be right.

A further hazard, of course, is the visiting vandal who wreaks his mindless evil on the creatures within the zoo from time to time. He tends to prefer the more defenceless creatures – wallabies or penguins (only yesterday I post-mortemed another rock-hopper penguin at Chessington Zoo, the second in one week to have his skull bashed flat by some brave marauder) – or easy targets like crocodiles. After being hit on the head with a five-pound lump of rock, a fine old alligator at Belle Vue didn't eat another thing in the nineteen remaining months of his life. We raised the depressed fracture of his skull and set the shattered pieces of bone with superglue bought from Woolworths, but although the skull healed satisfactorily there was nothing we could do about the terrible damage to his little brain. And sometimes we find evidence of poisoners at work – a dolphin deliberately fed crystals of copper sulphate secreted in fish, slug-killer given to bears. Malicious doping, usually by means of barbiturates, has plagued Chester Zoo over the years and I'd had one major attack at Belle Vue. On that occasion cats of every sort – leopards, tigers, pumas and lions – had been affected, the tigers most profoundly of all. It isn't too difficult to recognise the signs of barbiturate poisoning and I'd been able to confirm the diagnosis by having blood samples analysed at Newmarket by the laboratory people who specialise in spotting 'nobbled' horses. I hadn't been certain that the poisoning was deliberate: there was always the chance that the cats had been fed meat innocently contaminated with drugs, perhaps a horse euthanased by a vet's injection and then sent to a knackerman who forgot that the horsemeat would still contain the euthanasia drug. When the Newmarket lab reported that they'd been able to pinpoint the exact kind of barbiturate, butobarbitone, I was rather disturbed. There is no sort of butobarbitone injection that a vet might use on any animal for either anaesthesia or euthanasia, but there are plenty of butobarbitone sleeping pills around prescribed for humans. How could butobarbitone pills find their way, accidentally and in high numbers, into the meat used for feeding big cats?

We never solved that question, but all the animals recovered – and that's where the strong coffee came in. Given as an enema three times a day, it had helped immensely in earlier cases. It was a safe and lasting stimulant and it combated dehydration and kidney failure; since starting what one venerable head keeper had christened my 'Nescafé-up-the-arse' therapy, I hadn't lost a single case of drug intoxication in large felines. I had a feeling as I raced through the wooded Crown Land that lies between my home and the safari park that the Windsor cheetahs might be another case of barbiturate poisoning. I'd give them coffee till it came out of their ears. Of all the big cats, the cheetah is the most delicate and likeliest to die at the slightest excuse.

I turned into the park entrance, flashed my headlights at the girl in the cashbox and drove straight through to the cheetah reserve. With all the visitors about it would be quicker going in at the exit lock-gates to avoid the slow queue through the tiger and lion sections. As usual, drivers hooted and gesticulated wildly when they saw me going in the wrong direction against the traffic flow.

Francis met me in the corner of the reserve where three animals now lay motionless. Some 'dancers' were still on the floor and other cheetahs walked slowly over the grass close by. Cheetahs are harmless creatures to work amongst, and even in the breeding season it isn't dangerous to walk through their big reserve or even enter one of the small inspection pens with them. There are no known cases of cheetahs attacking men and although they have big teeth, powerful jaws and long, non-retractable claws, they never use them on humans unless handled unwisely. They are nervy beasts and, I believe, suffer far more easily than do the other big cats from stress and the side-effects of stress in captivity; these delightful feline greyhounds demand space, privacy and meticulous attention to design when a zoological collection wishes to introduce them. Windsor's cheetah section is one of the best in Britain and it is even equipped with two cheery little Jack Russell terriers who guard the indoor quarters against rodent night-visitors after dark and patrol the ditches and fence-line during the day.

'They seem to fall into three groups,' said Francis as we stood and looked around us. 'The ones that are flat out, the ones doing this staggering dance and a few that are just a wee bit rocky on their hind-legs. Also there appear to be others that are completely unaffected.' He pointed to one large male racing under the beech trees in fruitless pursuit of a wood pigeon that looked likely to make it into the branches.

I knelt down by one of the unconscious animals, felt for the femoral pulse in the warm groin and peered at the eyes. The mouth looked an unpleasant lilac colour and breathing was weak and shallow. A dancing cheetah brushed my back and I turned to watch it swing away. The feline fandango was in reality a form of ataxia, partial loss of control over the limb muscles. Francis was right: the animals did display three different clinical pictures more or less, but there were differences of degree. The dilating pupils of the eyes convinced me that my earlier guess looked likely to be proved right. The animals were doped and a barbiturate was the odds-on culprit.

I called over the warden for the cheetah section. 'When were these animals last fed?' I asked him.

'About five hours ago.'

'Were they absolutely normal before then?'

'Right as ninepence. I'll bet my life on that, Doctor.'

'What kind of meat did you give them?'

'To tell the truth, I don't know.'

'Don't know. What do you mean, you don't know?' Was the man daft or blind, I thought, and the irritation showed in my voice.

'Well, I gave a group of them a whole carcass, and I'm pretty sure that these sick ones are that group.'

'Yes, yes, but what kind of bloody carcass, for God's sake?'

The warden shrugged his shoulders and puffed out his cheeks. He gave a small embarrassed laugh. 'I really don't know, Doctor. It had no head on and no skin. Just a skinned carcass, fresh delivered by the knackerman this morning.'

'How big was this mysterious corpse? Goat, donkey, carthorse, cow, Loch Ness Monster?'

He stretched out his arms. 'About so long. Good-quality meat, I thought. Around seventy pounds weight altogether.'

'Were there four legs and what were the feet like?'

The warden pondered for a while. He was certain that the carcass had consisted of four legs, a trunk and a neck, but neither he nor his assistant could remember seeing the feet. We looked over the ground where the cheetahs had been fed. Only blood smears remained on the grass and a few slivers of bone. The cats wouldn't have eaten a hoof or well-developed cow's foot, but they might have relished a pig's trotter or the soft horn of a still-born calf. My guess was that the carcass without a name probably came minus its feet. So how to identify the species now?

'There is one thing I'm pretty sure of,' said the warden as I picked up an unrecognisable bone fragment. 'This group of cheetahs fed communally like they generally do on the carcass. Yellow Tag here and Blue Tag over there — he gestured towards the two deeply unconscious cats — stood side by side eating at the neck end. I can't recall the exact positions of all the others in the group but I think Clubfoot, who hardly seems affected at all, was at the opposite end of the body.'

All the cheetahs were easily identifiable. Many carried plastic ear-tags as part of the breeding record scheme instituted by the Smart family. Clubfoot was so named because of a distinctive enlargement of a front wrist joint that Francis and I had long ago X-rayed and found to be a chronic and incurable but apparently painless bone deformity.

If what the warden was saying was correct, it might be that the poison was concentrated or introduced into the carcass at one particular point, the neck. But even so, for so many animals to be affected the drug must have been distributed in some way throughout its tissues. I looked at the bit of bone in my hand: not only was I absolutely in the dark as to which species of animal it belonged to, I couldn't even tell what part of the skeleton it was from. It could have been a tail-tip or a bit of the skull. Putting it in my pocket, I got down to the business of trying to revive the narcotised cheetahs. 'Get those that can walk back to the night houses,' I told the warden. 'The worst ones we'll carry in the cars.'

Very soon we had all the patients indoors and I began the anti-barbiturate treatment. Francis carefully pumped the strong coffee he'd prepared into the rear end of the almost comatose animals. After taking blood for poison analysis, I squatted at their heads, giving injections of doxapram into the foreleg vein and warm saline under the skin over their ribs. The depressed breathing was causing the lilac colour of the mouth that signified cyanosis, but as soon as the doxapram circulated round to the brain things should improve. Sure enough, I saw the chest expand more strongly as the drug hit the right spot.

With deeply anaesthetised animals lying on their sides there is always the risk that the underneath lung will become congested with blood through the action of gravity on a sluggish pulmonary circulation. That had happened to me years before with Mary, a Belle Vue elephant with tooth trouble, and I had lost her from hypostatic pneumonia that had set in rapidly on the heels of the lung congestion. Cheetahs being infinitely more easy to handle than elephants, I instructed one of the cheetah keepers to stay with the doped animals and turn them over every twenty minutes until, as I always say in such circumstances with big cats, 'you are in danger of getting bitten or clawed by the beast as it wakes up.' Deeply narcotised tigers may need this regular turning for up to two days and nights.

There was nothing more to be done for the moment. The injections would need repeating every six or seven hours. By tomorrow I would know if we had won.

I went with Francis to look at the other animals. None of the cheetahs which had fed separately from the affected group was showing any signs of doping, nor were any of the lions or tigers. The drugged meat was almost certainly confined to the one carcass consumed by my patients, but just to be on the safe side, I asked the keepers to use the remainder of the stock of beef, sheep and pig meat only for feeding the old male lions. If there was any more spiked food around, they were tougher, and to be honest less valuable, than the cheetahs or tigers. Francis would order more meat from the knackerman and also ask him if he could throw any light onto the mystery of the nature and origin of the headless carcass.

The regular treatment of the doped cheetahs continued. The doxapram injections, which broke through the cloud of barbiturate that was numbing the brain cells and stimulated breathing, needed topping up. The working of the kidneys needed frequent monitoring and the amount of saline injection adjusted, but by the following day the position was much improved. Only two cheetahs were still on the danger list but even they were beginning to come round. I could tell this by the way the ears would flick automatically if I dropped a little cold water into them, and by the fact that they drew their legs back ever so slightly when I nipped them on the delicate skin between a pair of toes. To my delight one cheetah even gave a feeble growl of disapproval, even though still unconscious, when I prodded its anus with a pencil-point to test the reaction of the sphincter muscle.

Francis had been in contact with the knackerman but as I feared, he couldn't give us any useful information. Many dozens of animals went through his charnel-house every day – sides of beef that hadn't passed muster for human consumption, cattle struck by lightning, ponies destroyed after road accidents, sows dying in the process of giving birth, sheep seriously worried by dogs, even the occasional zoo animal that had died of disease or old age. It wasn't possible to say what or even how many kinds of animals had made up the half-ton assignment of meat feed delivered to Windsor.

It looked as though we would never get to the bottom of the puzzle. Like some near-perfect murder case, the body had totally disappeared except that in this case the body had been the weapon or at least the vehicle of death. The I remembered the bit of bone I had picked up on the previous day. I rooted round in my pocket and looked at it again. Still I hadn't a clue as to what animal the little splinter might have belonged to. How to identify it, if at all? I knew that a forensic laboratory could use the precipitin test to establish the specific origin of a speck of tissue or blood, so I decided to try the anatomists at Cambridge: perhaps someone in Professor Harrison's department of veterinary anatomy would be able to recognise something about the structure of the bony morsel that would give it a name. I put it in an envelope with a covering letter and sent it by the next post. Meanwhile a phone call had come in from the Newmarket laboratory – the cheetah blood was strongly positive for pentobarbitone.

As the days went by, the need for doxapram became less but the importance of fluid to combat dehydration of the doped and undrinking cheetahs increased. When the animals were compos mentis enough to cause trouble I gave their saline transfusions in the special crush-cages that are fitted to two of the 'hospital' dens in their house. Bit by bit the cats returned to normality and when they were finally steady on their feet and able to eat and drink again, Francis and his team could relax.

170

The Cambridge University anatomists came up trumps and coinciding with the end of the cheetah therapy came a letter with a report on the bone fragment: it was part of a bovine upper foreleg. I discussed the result with Francis and our conclusions were far from satisfactory. We knew from the warden's report that the carcass had been a whole one and not very large. Now found to be bovine, it must have been a large calf. The fact that the cheetahs feeding on the neck end had been worst affected and those at the rear end least so might indicate that the barbiturate had been injected into the calf's jugular vein. If there had been a leakage around the needle injection site, a not uncommon occurrence, the drug would have accumulated in fairly high concentration in the neck tissues and remained there long enough to poison whatever fed on the calf after its death. One big query remained: why would anyone inject a calf in the jugular with a barbiturate? Dogs, cats and sometimes horses are humanely euthanised by veterinarians using intravenous barbiturates, but I have never heard of a calf being destroyed in this way. A farmer wanting to have a calf killed would take it to the slaughter-house, where a humane killer would be used to avoid spoiling the meat.

Another possibility was that the animal had been given an intravenous shot of pentobarbitone as an anaesthetic for some operation, perhaps to correct a hernia or for castration, and had died under anaesthesia. But again this seemed highly unlikely: barbiturates had been used years before for anaesthetising cattle, but had had several disadvantages and had been superseded by much more satisfactory and efficient drugs. I couldn't imagine any veterinarian in this day and age using the fairly long-acting pentobarbitone, a drug that wasn't easily cleared from the animal's system and whose original antidote was no longer manufactured, on a calf needing surgical attention. The knackerman could not recall picking up any calves said to have succumbed during an operation, although it isn't usual for such information to reach the knackerman in any case: he simply picks up the deceased and hurries off.

The third possibility was the most worrying of all: malicious introduction of the drug into the carcass. Could someone have stuffed a handful of Nembutal sleeping capsules into the open neck-end? It would have been possible, although security in the park was at a high level and the meat store was deep within the big cat reserves. I knew all the wardens and keepers and couldn't believe that any one of them would have done such an insane thing, yet it surely could not have been an outsider unless someone had tampered with the meat before it came to the safari park.

The mystery was insoluble and so it has remained to this day. No more barbiturate poisonings have occurred at Windsor and whenever I drive through the cheetah reserve at the park and see those big cats lying elegant as sphinxes under the trees or chasing the feed-truck expectantly, I always return to wondering: how did the knock-out drug get into that one hapless calf?

Although by now I had been living in the South almost long enough to become accustomed to its commuter hybrids, chocolate-box scenery and watery beer, I still valued the link with the North provided by Belle Vue Zoo in Manchester. I had started my practice with exotic animals there and it occupied a special place in my affections, so it was with a real sense of personal loss that I heard the announcement that it was to close down. The famous gardens, established in the reign of King William IV, had come to the end of the road.

When the news first broke, I could not believe it. Manchester without Bell Vue Zoo? The place where I'd gone as a boy to see the only tigon on exhibition in the whole world, where within its walls even now stood animal houses modelled on Mogul pavilions, where the first alligators to lay eggs in a British zoo had lived, where up until only a few years before a visitor might find the best aquarium, great ape house and tropical river house in the country? The major collection of animals that had been rated one of England's top three zoos as late as the mid-1960s, where I had learned through a million moments of heartache, frustration, incomprehension and occasional exhilaration the groundwork of my craft, where I'd seen my first elephant dissected, knocked out my first gorilla, made a wooden leg for a flamingo and a new plastic tendon for a hamstrung wallaby, delivered my first infant monkey by Caesarian and resuscitated new-born polar bear twins – Belle Vue? Putting up the shutters?

The truth of the matter was that the old zoo had stopped ageing gracefully and begun to show extensive signs of senile decay. Lack of exercise and the right sort of nursing in recent years had brought on incurable economic arthritis, an ailment that particularly menaces the senior citizens of the zoo world, the classic city animal parks.

There had been many contributory factors: the state of some of the buildings, which had been neglected for too long and would by now have been prohibitively expensive to replace; the cost of maintaining a large collection on grounds which possessed virtually no grassland; competition from the new wave of zoos that had begun in the mid-1960s, the safari parks and country parks that gave folk an opportunity to travel out into the countryside rather than travel in to one of the most seedy and dilapidated areas of an industrial city; and above all the loss of a sense of its own purpose. Belle Vue was not alone in failing to adapt to a world which had rapidly, under the important influences of television and rising public awareness of what wildlife is all about, changed the ground rules for animal exhibition. The zoo had never been able to grasp fully the new need to educate more than to entertain. Nor had it concentrated on the things that can be done well in cities and discarded displays better left to the new rural parks like Longleat and Marwell which possessed a coherent and up-to-date set of aims.

As a general rule the movement of big business into the zoo 'industry', which began around 1970, was to prove a slow but deadly poison for many important collections – and it is a lethal process which has not yet run its full course. Companies with spare capital were looking for 'diversification' with high hopes of abundant returns, and the mushrooming leisure field was to be the happy hunting ground. Zoos were part of the leisure field, exactly like bingo halls, bowling alleys and funfairs – so grab a piece of the action and buy yourself a zoo. Besides, wouldn't the wildlife dimension, in among the one-armed bandits, the self-service counters, the roulette wheels and the discothèques, add a touch of class to the company image? Yes, indeed, was the unanimous response of the accountants, financiers and entrepreneurs who ran the companies.

Big business arrived in the zoo world with two fatal misconceptions: one, that every animal man is by nature uncommercial, a sort of bucolic innocent who is unlikely to be able to master the finer points of a Post Office Savings Bank account; and two, that everyone knows the basics about animals. Doesn't every banker, every tinker, tailor and candlestick-maker have a budgie or a pet corgi or a polo pony or a goldfish? Doesn't everyone watch David Attenborough on TV, read *Ring of Bright Water* and have a camel ride when they're on holiday in the Canaries? Everyone likes animals, so can't anyone supervise the running of a zoo? I have been regularly and unfailingly amazed by the chairmen, secretaries, accountants and legal advisors of large organisations newly arrived on the zoo scene who really do believe that, because they hobby-farm a handful of goats on five acres of land at their country cottage, they are qualified to lay down the law on the feeding of Malayan tapirs or the treatment of Tasmanian devils. I remember well that when one zoo with which I was associated was taken over by just such a company, the Chairman, a Tory MP with a safe rural seat and some cattle on the side although not a professional farmer, lectured me with great pomposity on the maintenance of exotic animals including a killer whale, the first he had ever seen and which came with the purchase.

Such organisations dashed into the zoos and safari parks putting hacks, has-beens, whizz-kids or failures drafted from other parts of their empires into the driving seats: 'Simpkins doesn't seem to fit in the Bingo Division and he's not got the head for figures that we need in Casinos; let's give him a spell at the *Zoo* until there's a vacancy at Executive Grade 3(a) level on the Hotel side.' After all isn't 'management' a self-contained, catholic profession? Don't ask what is to be managed; just go and manage it.

Worse still, big business introduced into the zoo world a pathogen more virulent than foot-and-mouth or anthrax spores — the all-powerful accountant. After all, ran the argument, the techniques for the financial management of any organisation are essentially the same, are they not, irrespective of what field it is operating in? It is all a question of systematic application of Good Business Management principles to the Units. Ah, what neat, scientific, precise order that word conjures up! And zoos are self-evidently composed of Units, lovely units for the accountant to play with, comprising groups of buildings, groups of animals or, if Your Accountancy so desires, individual animal 'units'. Any company accountant worth his pocket calculator quickly saw that zoos could be looked at in just the same way as restaurants, amusement arcades or bingo halls.

They were wrong.

It may seem unnecessary to say it to you, dear reader, but tigers and turtles and touracos are totally different from vending machines and roller coasters and night clubs. It took some time, as far as big business was concerned, for the penny to drop.

At Belle Vue distinguished zoo-men who were responsible for the care of the animals, such as Raymond Legge, never had a seat on the park board. As a general rule staff with real knowledge and experience of wild animals were never appointed to levels higher than middle management in the newly-arrived companies. And Belle Vue was by no means as bad in that respect as were some others, where major decisions involving the animals, including the actual design and erection of some animal housing, were sometimes made without any advice from animal people. The ultimate fate of the beasts lay in the hands of lawyers, financiers, speculators and the faceless 'manager'.

We became used to being asked daft questions like how much illness should be budgeted for in the next financial period and could we estimate which would prove less expensive: poor-quality, cheaper foodstuffs plus increased incidence of disease versus better, dearer foodstuffs plus less sickness. One zoo's accountant actually agonised to me over the difficulty of quantifying the financial yield of an elephant to set against its cost of hay, grain, fruit and winter heating. 'We really must find some way of calculating the productivity per animal,' he moaned. 'I can see what the sealions,

175

riding camels and pony rides produce in terms of cash because of the extra internal charges to the visitors. But those elephants! Nothing but a drain on our running expenses, bloody great guts full of food and nothing to show for it.'

He meant, I suppose, on the ledger in neatly typed, impassive numbers. What was the fellow doing – in a zoo!

The error was not in applying the profit motive to zoos. Zoological parks can't be divided into 'commercial' and 'non-commercial' (by implication, superior) operations; an elephant, whether it is in Belle Vue or Regent's Park, may scoff as much as 600 lbs of vegetable matter per day, every day of the year. The cash to buy that food has to be generated somehow, and the generation of cash is in all British zoos an almost totally 'commercial' process. The problem arises in the concept of profit – what it is, what it should be and how it should be used.

I am not by any means suggesting that a better classification should be into 'non-profit-making' (i.e. good) or 'profit-making' (i.e. bad) zoos; major influences in high-quality zoological innovation in the 1960s and 1970s had been people like Jimmy Chipperfield (Longleat, Woburn and the father of the safari park principle), Pentland Hick (Flamingo Park, and the pioneer of marine mammal exhibition) and the Smart family (Windsor Safari Park). Their companies not only made profits but also provided the best in animal management both in front of and behind the scenes. So why did they succeed so brilliantly while the bigger, more formally organised companies, riding in at their heels with such self-esteem, tended sooner rather than later to bite the dust?

I am sure that the people from the big companies, even the accountants, would have said they liked animals, but liking just isn't enough by a long chalk if animal-keeping of any sort is to be conducted successfully. A feeling for, an excitement with, an empathy towards living creatures, not necessarily a degree in zoology or veterinary medicine, is what you need. That is what the Chipperfields, Hicks, Smarts and others like Durrell in Jersey, Knowles at Marwell and Mottershead at Chester had in abundance. The organisation men of the big business concerns did not. It was the central reason for their failure. A good zoo puts its animals first, the visitors respond and profits may follow. Reverse the order and put profits first, the animals come under all sorts of pressure, the displays suffer, visitors dwindle and a bad zoo becomes worse.

When Belle Vue finally closed its gates, Ray Legge's successor, Peter Grayson, was zoo superintendent. To him fell the melancholy task of disposing of the stock, a job that took him almost one and a half years following the closure. Finding suitable new homes for some of the older inmates was almost impossible. Over the past ten years the British zoo world has become increasingly self-sufficient in stocking itself with animals. Many species now breed with ease, and in the case of some creatures such as tigers, lions, pumas, bears and various kinds of hoofed animal there is a positive over-population problem. In 1965 a lion fetched a price of between £250 and £300. Nowadays it isn't worth one-fiftieth of that. With a properly-constructed box to transport it in costing perhaps £150, the container has become far more valuable than the contents! Sadly, in death the noble big cat regains his value because of the lively market in lion skins, and a dead adult male will bring what his live relative did in 1965.

We didn't get cracking with animal contraception early enough. At Windsor our lion-breeding programme has always been carefully geared to the demand for cubs in new parks at home and abroad, and we have even exported Windsor lion cubs back to Africa! At the peak of our lion 'farming' we were hand-rearing from the moment of birth a hundred lion cubs per year with zero mortality rate up to weaning. When the demand from suitable homes slackened (the Smarts' firm policy was never to provide cubs as exotic pets or for other gimmicky purposes), we started controlling the fertility of the lionesses, each of which was identified by a coloured plastic ear-tag. First we used the 'Pill', administered in their meat, but later we found it more efficient to inject them in the Windsor treatment cages with long-acting progesterone. Nowadays we use an even better method, simply slipping a small porous plastic tube containing solid contraceptive chemical under the skin of an anaesthetised big cat. I make a careful drawing in my records showing where the implant is buried (I try, for example, to place it where two stripes meet on the side of a tiger) so that the process can be reversed by retrieval of the implant should we want to re-start reproduction at any time. Rarely now do I remove the ovaries of a female or vasectomise a male, as I much prefer to leave our future options open with the safe and simple reversible techniques.

But overall the baby boom in many species has caught the zoos off balance and some creatures, male llamas being a chronic example, are a drug on the market. That was why Peter Grayson had to scour Europe and beyond to find places in zoos for all the Belle Vue animals to which he was as deeply attached as I was, even though he had only been associated with the zoo for about four years. Old friends that I'd wrestled with, puzzled over, been chastised by and acted as family doctor to since they'd first arrived or been born in the zoo were gradually dispersed.

The sombre exodus took the form of a trickle rather than a flood. Each time I visited the zoo to do my routine checks another few of my long-standing furry or feathered cronies had disappeared. It was always the same: they were moved out, leaving uneaten food in their mangers, familiar droppings on the floor and skid-marks in the sand or sawdust. Their pens, many of which hadn't been unoccupied since 1836, were never cleaned out after they'd gone. Quickly, so very quickly as if Nature was made hasty by embarrassment, the weeds and the mould, the wind and the rust and the sparrows moved into the silent houses so that after only a few weeks it was difficult to accept that these chilly clanging rooms, stagnant pools and doors jammed ajar had so recently held the cacophony, the aromas, the blood-warmth of jungles and swamps and steppes.

Some of my old patients did well by the break-up. Twiggie, one of the elephants, went to Amersfoort in Holland, where I still keep an eye on her, and the superb Madrid Zoo acquired our big alligators. Others fared less well. Poor old Hercules the hippo,* a

* See *Zoovet.*

178

favourite adversary of mine and undisputed king of the tropical house, went to Cleethorpes, narrowly escaped being euthanased when the zoo there folded shortly after his arrival and no-one seemed to want him, and by the skin of his enormous teeth found a new berth at Dudley, another city zoo soon to face problems of its own. He died shortly after.

The pair of gorillas, Suzy and Jo-Jo, whom I'd attended since they were infants, were tragically split up. Suzy went to Bristol and Jo-Jo to Chester. Jo-Jo, by now a strapping mature 'silver-back', hadn't been there very long before he fell ill and died. I know it is grossly unscientific and totally out of character for me to state this, but I firmly believe that the stress of separation from his mate after all those years, together with the new environment, played a major part in his death. I do not for a moment doubt the pathologist's report but I bet my bottom dollar that Jo-Jo and Suzy would still be living together as happy as Larry if Belle Vue hadn't closed. Some of the chimps, including one I had operated on for a chest-wall tumour when it was a baby, I saw recently in a travelling circus.

Although it was kept a secret from me and most other folk at the time to avoid bad publicity for the company which intended to continue operating the non-zoological parts of the Belle Vue park, some of the animals were destroyed when Peter found it absolutely impossible even to give them away to people qualified to look after them properly. When in the latter days some of the snakes escaped from their vivaria almost as if they were making a desperate dash for freedom, the company bulldozed the reptile house flat – just in case. All the other houses were left to moulder away. It was an atrociously sad time.

As the animal numbers diminished so too was the staff progressively cut back. Matt Kelly, the doyen of British zoo head keepers and the man who'd taught me many a way with animals as student and tyro veterinarian, retired. Eventually Peter was down to one elephant, Ellie May, and one keeper to take care of her until she too went through the gates. The months went by. Belle Vue Zoo continued to exist: one superintendent, one keeper, one zoo vet, one good old Indian elephant. The four of us met regularly in the Victorian elephant house, and Ellie May would chomp apples and watch us with glistening eyes as we discussed her future. One thing became very clear: nobody wanted Ellie May either to buy or as a gift.

As the second winter since the zoo officially closed approached, the company was viewing with little relish the prospect of heating bills and extra food for the sole survivor. What was to be done? It came to me through the grapevine that the chairman of the company was concerned about the situation. If no home could be found for the elephant, then there might be pressure on us that it should be euthanased – the Manchester zoo would finally be laid to rest. How ironic: what had begun for me all those years ago in this very same elephant house, when as a student I had watched the awful enormity of my first post-mortem on Chota, another elephant,* would have come full circle. Belle Vue had begun for me in the death of an elephant and might end in the same way. But whereas Chota had been painfully crippled with osteo-arthritis, Ellie May was as fit and lively as a fiddle. Nothing would induce me to sign her death warrant for the sake of company tidiness. I didn't like keeping her alone in the great house that had once been alive with elephants, hippos, parrots and people, but I'd rather that than kill her, even if the company had to purchase hay, bread, cereal, fruit, vegetables and the gallons of Ribena that we used in the cold weather, as well as heating oil, for the next ten winters. Peter and I were in full agreement over the matter.

The second winter came and still Ellie May kept the zoo alive. Then one day Peter telephoned me with some great news. Rotterdam Zoo had agreed to take Ellie May and pay her transport costs! We were highly delighted; Rotterdam has a fine reputation among European zoos and their facilities and expertise are second to none.

'Hanne, it's going to be OK,' I said when I put down the receiver. 'The Belle Vue elephant has got a home to go to! The final exit, thank God, is going to be a dignified one.'

* See *Zoovet*.

'Fantastisch! See, I told you there was nothing to worry about!' She looked as elated as I was.

Hanne fetched the bottle of Polish vodka and we drank a toast to Ellie May and the last act in the life of the great zoo that had done so much for me. Little did we suspect as we sipped the Wyborowa that Belle Vue hadn't finished with me yet and that the ghost of Chota, dead over a quarter of a century, was still unexorcised.

Ellie May was an opinionated elephant who had always held firm opinions about what she did and did not like. Among the former were her keeper, brown ale, Swiss rolls, mice (lots of them lived in the elephant house and could be seen most mornings actually dining with Ellie May at her pile of fruit and cereals) and umbrellas, quite a few of which she had snatched, chewed up, swallowed and successfully passed through her intestines. The latter comprised onions, vets with hypodermic syringes, and sloping surfaces. Many elephants are disinclined to go up ramps or artificial inclines of any sort and they're very sensitive to anything that gives or wobbles slightly underfoot. Perhaps you'd feel the same way if you weighed up to ten tonnes! Ellie May had proved to be rather stubborn about loading ramps in the past. Maybe, elephant-like, she never forgot some treacherous surface that she'd come across in her youth. Peter decided to take no chances and asked me about the wisdom of tranquillising her slightly for the loading.

'I'll take her straight out of the elephant house with the keeper on one side and me on the other,' he said. 'The truck is a big new one and we'll have it backed right up to the door with the ramp solidly wedged by straw bales. We'll begin at first light when there's no-one about and nothing to distract her. Straight out, up the ramp and in. Do you think she'll need a sedative?'

'Certainly not a sedative,' I replied. 'The one thing we don't want is any hint of grogginess. A drunken elephant or one that knuckles over on the ramp and decides to have a nap would be disastrous.'

'She's a headstrong old love, though. One refusal and we might as well pack up for a year at the least. And if she decides to, she's capable of side-stepping the ramp and making for the city centre with bits of the elephant house and what remains of the big new elephant truck round her neck!'

I had seen Ellie May doing her own thing with slopes. On one occasion, filming a documentary for Southern Television and with Peter riding her mahout-style, she had repeatedly run amok on reaching a certain concrete incline in the zoo grounds, dashing into the trees and wiping her rider off against the branches as easily and brutally as she would rid herself of an irritating tick. The solution might be to give her a small dose of tranquilliser by injection. Just a little, to clear the mind of elephantine anxieties.

'I'll give her a wee drop of acepromazine half an hour before we start loading,' I told Peter. 'Get everything prepared and I'll see you at six o'clock in the morning. Oh, and get some brown ale and half a dozen Swiss rolls.'

Ellie May's last day at Belle Vue dawned grey, dry and cold. When I arrived the elephant truck was in position. Its great length had been painstakingly introduced into the small yard behind the elephant house by innumerable to-ings and fro-ings of the powerful motor. The ramp was solidly in place at the threshold of the big doors. The ramp sides were stoutly fenced and there wasn't a chink between them and the door edges. Inside I found Peter and the keeper quietly giving breakfast to Ellie May and the odd early-rising mouse. The elephant was in a kindly mood and tolerated my injection into her buttocks with nothing more than a lazy cuff to my head from her trunk. Half an hour later Peter and the keeper each with one hand on an ear and the other hand laden with Swiss roll chunks, and with a bucket of brown ale standing in the front of the elephant truck, led Ellie May out of her house for the last time, down the passage towards the doorway. I followed quietly behind. She moved perfectly with no sign of agitation and not a hint of doziness. She arrived placidly at the foot of the ramp, Peter murmured words of encouragement and proffered a large piece of the sugary cake, her trunk reached forwards as the sensitive nostrils picked up the whiff of Samuel Smith's Old Brewery Strong on the morning air, and she started steadily up the slope.

182

At the top of the ramp, and with half her body already within the truck, Ellie May changed her mind. Going smoothly and steadily into reverse, she backed out again and to our dismay lay down on the ramp.

The next few hours were sheer hell. We pushed and pulled, cajoled and pleaded, enticed and shouted. More men were sent for to heave and lever, the truck's own winch was carefully used until Ellie May flicked a leg effortlessly and stripped the gears. It was all to no avail. The more we attempted to 'daddy' her around on the ramp, the worse her position became. Manoeuvring the truck in the confined space brought half a wall down and fractured steel plates on the vehicle itself. I blew in her ear as hard as I could and gave her stimulant injections. Zero. Little by little Ellie May wriggled herself onto her side, but with her giant legs splayed out awkwardly. A tractor and then a crane were summoned and proved useless; Ellie May wasn't prepared to give us one iota of help. There was no sign of injury and she wasn't in pain or distress. She simply seemed to have decided not to go, not under any circumstances.

By the time evening came I was deeply alarmed. I had begun to detect the first signs of physiological complications arising in the spreadeagled colossus that lay amidst the rubble of a futile day's labour, surrounded by sweating, exhausted men and palely lit by flashlights. There were fluid sounds in the lungs, the pulse of the great femoral artery was faster and less full, and the normally salmon-pink mouth was now more pale. I gave circulation-supporting drugs by injection straight into the ear-veins and sent for hay bales, thick rugs and a bottle of brandy to warm her.

Peter was ashen-faced and almost dropping on his feet. 'What do you think?' he asked. 'Isn't this . . .' He couldn't finish the sentence but I knew exactly what he was thinking.

'Let's pack it in for tonight,' I said. 'There's nothing more to be done for the moment. Maybe with a rest during the night she'll pull herself together and make fools of us all by getting up as nimbly as you please.'

Both of us knew that was bullshit. I went over to Rochdale to sleep at my parents' house. Peter stayed up with Ellie May.

As dawn broke the following morning I went back to Belle Vue. As I knew I would, I found Ellie May still lying in a heap like a gigantic grey frog. Her posture had put pressure on her internal organs and her lungs were now in severe trouble. Hypostatic pneumonia was established and the heart was failing.

There was nothing else for it. 'She must be euthanased,' I told Peter.

He nodded, his face haggard and covered with greasy grey elephant dust. 'Will you do it?' he asked quietly.

'No. Send for a marksman to do it. Point-blank. Heart-shot.'

I have never felt more desolate. Fate had dealt me a preposterous, satanic hand. It was the end of a tragic full circle, yet one which had encompassed some of the happiest moments of my life. At my beginning there had been Chota. Then there had been Mary, dying of this same hypostatic pneumonia under anaesthetic in the days before I had the reversible modern drugs. And now at my ending with Belle Vue there was this sickening mess. I have never personally destroyed an elephant. If Ellie May was to go, she must go at the hand of someone else, but someone reliable. Peter was well acquainted with firearms and we had plenty of weapons in the zoo armoury, but I knew he felt as I did.

A marksman from the local gun club who lived nearby was sent for. When he arrived I chalked a circle on the skin over Ellie May's heart and made some excuse about needing to make arrangements with the knackerman. I went to my old dispensary inside the elephant house to make the call. When the bang eventually came it seemed so extraordinarily loud that it must have wakened half of Manchester.

Presently I went back, checked Ellie May's heart with my stethoscope to make absolutely sure and then slipped quietly away. I wasn't interested in doing a post-mortem this time. That was the way the world, at Belle Vue, ended.

Every few months or so I like to drive through the deserted zoo at Manchester. It's difficult to know precisely why. It pleases me that the park gateman, new to the job since the zoo closed, always waves me through immediately with a 'Right you are, sir, carry on' when I wind down the car window and say, 'Good morning, it's the vet' just like I always used to. Maybe there are still tigers and giraffes somewhere in there as far as he is concerned. There certainly are for me as I walk through the dilapidated buildings, noting some ancient oryx droppings here, a pile of sunflower seed husks discarded by one of my long-gone macaws over there, a familiar piece of rope-netting in a corner of the monkey house through which I was once well and truly bitten, a tree now in full blossom where the leopard holed up after it escaped, and a thousand other things that bring the whole glorious gallimaufry back to life.

10

An unusual lull of a few days in the normally pressing demands of the telephone and telex gave me a breather during which I was able to take my mind off Ellie May and Belle Vue by catching up with my writing – and my cooking. I was finishing a small book on cooking for pets that had been commissioned by the BBC, a laborious task with every meal from Marrowbone à la Marmaduke, through slimming dishes for tubby dogs, to economy cook-ups for the pets of OAPs having to be prepared and tested. Tsar Nicholas I's chef de cuisine at St Petersburg in 1829 may have concocted a divine bortsch and had the lightest of hands in beating the blini mixture, but the appearance, smell and taste of the dish that he prepared daily for his Imperial master's cat struck me as repellent in the extreme. Lenin, my own cat-about-town and feline bon viveur, seemed to agree after I had presented for his approval a dish of caviar poached in champagne, together with minced dormouse, woodcock's egg, butter, hare's blood, cream, chervil and Sukhumi cheese. He gave the moggy equivalent of the thumbs down by shaking a paw over the khaki-coloured mess and stalking off, looking rather peeved. Mind you, I had had to use lumpfish roe, minced chicken, a bantam egg and Edam as substitutes for the best Beluga, dormouse, woodcock egg and unobtainable Asiatic Russian cheese, but the champagne was vintage Taittinger and the cream from our milkman is as thick and delicious as anything the Romanovs might have enjoyed.

My own culinary ambition has always been to create the perfect shellfish sauce for my favourite form of Italian pasta, spaghetti alla vongole. Essentially a simple dish, it nevertheless hides subtleties which many a ristorante misses, and the quest to bring this ambrosia into being has given me hours of delicious relaxation. The vongole itself, that is the Italian clam and its American counterpart, are feeble creatures and not up to a starring role. Cockles harvested off the north Lancashire coast have them licked for taste and bite. But then I experimented with the plump cockle that is found on the south coast of England near Littlehampton. This sublime mollusc is unquestionably the Mohammed Ali or Maria Callas of vongole sauce-making: it has class. Get them alive if possible and fatten them overnight in the way my grandmother taught me by putting them in a bucket of salt, water and finest oatmeal. If the elephant is my favourite vertebrate, the cockle, may it rest in peace, is my best-loved invertebrate, although it is unlikely ever to enlist as one of my exotic patients. Nevertheless, when dolphin-catching in Florida, I once opened a large number of molluscs taken from waters contaminated by the Greater Miami sewer outfall and found over forty per cent of them to be afflicted by cancer.

With Lenin blackballing any question of even one Guide Michelin rosette for the poor Tsar's effort, I turned to the next experiment on my list – Felix's Fancy, a ragout of cods' roe and sweetbreads. Hanne popped her head round the kitchen door, surveyed forlornly the shambles that is the hallmark of my most inspired cooking and wrinkled her nose. It was probably the pan of lungs and spleen bubbling away happily on the stove in preparation for the Crufts Meat Loaf Extraordinaire.

'Liliana is on the phone from Madrid. It's the pandas again,' she told me. I took the receiver off the wall with a sticky hand. 'Ola, Liliana, que tal?'

Liliana wasn't in the mood for our usual preliminary banter about whether the Falkland Islands sea elephants are Argentinian or British or about who are the prettiest, the girls of Buenos Aires or the mesticos of Rio. 'David, Chang-Chang looks bad. Today he has had much mucus again but, for the first time, he is also vomiting. His weight is down to eighty kilos. Can you come at once?'

This was the crunch. The panda's symptoms which Andrew had first described to me by phone while I was in Abu Dhabi had proved as sinister as I'd feared. The animal would have to be thoroughly examined and that meant immobilising him far more completely than was possible with the crush-cage. A general anaesthetic was the only answer. And nobody then knew much about general anaesthesia in the giant panda.

'I'll catch the next plane, and get David Wild to fly down from Manchester as well. I'm going to look inside Chang-Chang's stomach.'

David was a skilled fibre-optic gastroscope operator, and essential for the more complicated procedures, using the long £6,000 Fujinon endoscope that Andrew and I had bought. He was busy at a hospital near Lancaster, turning a different model of endoscope through 180 degrees inside an unconscious middle-aged lady's duodenum so that it would proceed up her bile duct to have a look at a small tumour that was blocking it, when he received my message. As soon as the surgeons had garrotted the offending tumour with a fine wire loop passed through the endoscope, David left the operating theatre, washed and changed furiously and sprinted to his car. He had two hours to drive down the M6 to Ringway airport, catch the shuttle to Heathrow and pick up the last flight of the day to Madrid. Still smelling faintly of Lysol and halothane gas, he made it just before the aircraft door was closed.

'What's up then, maaster?' he gasped with deliberate exaggeration of his normal Yorkshire accent as he flopped down beside me. 'And tha' mun order me a double brandy when ah get back mi puff.'

In my hurry to get him down as fast as possible I had forgotten to say what we were going to Madrid for. It had been the same before on other emergencies when we'd travelled together to Germany, France, Spain and Panama; he sometimes hadn't even known which country we were going to until we'd met at the airport ticket desk. I outlined the potential problem to him as we sipped our brandy and he at once spotted the central dilemma.

'And how do you propose to knock t' bugger out then?' he enquired.

Quite so. How did one anaesthetise a giant panda for the first time? Or, more to the point, make sure it came round afterwards? I still carried the memory of the first monkey I had anaesthetised as a young vet, long before the special drugs for exotic animals were discovered; it had died promptly after my injection of Themalon, then one of the best preparations for dogs. I would have to make a decision and select something out of the Bag to do the trick. What was it to be? Etorphine, xylazine, barbiturates, Saffan, phencyclidine, ketamine, a gas like halothane or ether, one of the new experimental compounds such as tiletamine or a cocktail of two or more such potent chemicals? The names swarmed in my head like angry bees. By the time we were buckling our seat belts for landing in Spain, I still hadn't made up my mind.

It was not long after the New Year festivities, and there was frost in the air sharpening the familiar aroma of Madrid, a blend of toasted tobacco, furniture polish and chorizo sausage. Along the avenidas, the illuminated fountains spilled cataracts of light through the crisp evening gloom and Gregorian vespers flowed softly from the taxi radio as we drove through the Casa de Campo to the zoo. In the panda house kitchen we found Liliana, Antonio-Luis and the keepers huddled round the hot-plate, sipping strong black coffee from laboratory beakers.

A quick glance through the peep-hole at Chang-Chang confirmed Liliana's opinion. The male panda was continually retching and plainly suffering considerable abdominal pain which caused him to groan and shift restlessly in between the bouts of sickness. Ominously, I saw streaks of what looked like Turkish coffee grounds in his vomit — blood that had been turned brown through contact with stomach acids.

'Anaesthesia first thing in the morning,' I said to Liliana who had already recognised the significance of the 'coffee'.

'What anaesthetic will you use?'

'I'll know by morning. Let me sleep on it if I can.'

'What about the Panda Council?'

Ah, the Royal Panda Council! Its full title was actually much longer and sounded very grand. It had been appointed by the King to oversee on his behalf the maintenance of his two rare gifts. It consisted of several dukes, some city notables and a professor or two from the university as well as representatives of the zoo board, and in practice it did nothing at all. Theoretically the Council had to approve any and everything concerning the pandas, but from the beginning we had insisted that that would be utterly unacceptable in matters veterinary and the zoo directors, Dr Cerdan and Dr Celma, took all the day-to-day decisions out of the hands of the Council. We had developed a system of notifying the council after the fact.

'We'll send in a report but only after everything is over,' I replied.

'And what if . . . things go wrong?'

'We'll face the music then. But telling them about Chang-Chang's trouble now might invite interference and couldn't possibly produce any useful contributions towards the outcome. I'll take full responsibility.'

I hoped I sounded confident and cheerful to my colleagues. Within, I wondered what the reaction of King Juan Carlos and his Council would be if Chang-Chang did die under my anaesthetic. Had Torquemada's Inquisition any counterpart in modern Spain that could put heretic English veterinarians to the rack?

In my room at the Castellana later that night I found it impossible to sleep. I lay in bed with a balloon glass of Osborne brandy and the radio droning, carrying on a tense debate within my skull. Gas anaesthetics which could be gently applied little by little were out. It wasn't possible to hold a mask on Chang-Chang's face as if he were sitting peaceably in a dentist's chair, and using tubes on him would anyway mean the injection of some sort of knock-out chemical first in order to get the tubes down his windpipe. It all came back to the same question: what injectable anaesthetic would be safe and reliable in a giant panda? Nothing had been published, and the Chinese I'd visited in 1974 hadn't up to then revealed what, if anything, they knew about the subject. I knew well the incredibly powerful effects of minuscule quantities of etorphine on certain animals and remembered how it had killed humans and other primates. A teaspoonful was enough to stop a wild African bull elephant dead in its tracks, so what was the safe dose for a panda? Phencyclidine was long-acting and irreversible. Barbiturates were either too persistent or had to be given by intravenous injection only, and I couldn't guarantee getting a vein even in the crush-cage. Xylazine and Saffan were specialised drugs and again without reversing agents if anything went wrong. The new experimental drugs were far too chancy.

At last, as the wee small hours expanded into the greyer ones of dawn, I made up my mind. I would use a mixture of valium, the tranquilliser that I'd found safe in everything from chimp to hornbill, and ketamine, an anaesthetic that was quickly excreted by the mammalian body. Usually. The two were compatible in all the many exotic species I'd worked with over the years. I would gamble (pitiless but precise word) that it would be the same in the giant panda. Once the decision had been taken I fell into a deep, panda-free sleep that was soon interrupted by the room-waiter coming in with my tray of coffee and panecillos and drawing open the curtains.

By eight o'clock we were all assembled again in the panda house. Chang-Chang looked as miserable as ever as we tricked him into entering the crush-cage on the pretext that he was being allowed out into his paddock. Quickly but gently Antonio-Luis would turn the handle to compress him. While he was standing on his head during one of his marvellous feats of contortionism I jabbed my needle into his buttocks and pressed the syringe plunger. I had crossed the Rubicon.

One and a half minutes later, far more rapidly than I anticipated or approved of, Chang-Chang sank to his furry knees and fell unconscious. The cage door was opened and he was dragged out into the nearby room where I was to carry out the operation. To keep the panda's mouth open during the gastroscopy I needed some sort of gagging instrument. Tailor-made mouth-gags are sold for humans, dogs, cats, cattle, horses and other domestic animals. The market for panda mouth-gags being understandably small, no such instrument has yet been invented. I found, however, that a stainless steel retractor designed for holding human abdomens open served the purpose admirably, its opposing bars clipping neatly onto Chang-Chang's lower fang teeth.

David had meanwhile set up the electronic box of tricks that produces the intense beam of light, the water jet and the compressed air for the endoscope. A special camera stood ready to photograph everything we saw through the dual eye-pieces and there were sets of forceps, biopsy and cauterising instruments and Ryles' tubes to suck out samples of gastric juices. First I checked the panda's breathing and pulse and took a quantity of blood for analysis from a nice big vein that I found in his forearm, much in the same place that one lies in the dog, cat or lion. Prodding Chang-Chang's body with my fingers, I found him to be thin under his masking coat of thick fur. Then, after lubricating the endoscope thoroughly with surgical jelly, I began to introduce it over the back of the plump panda tongue and down his throat. David worked the remote controls, washing the lens clear of mucus and steering the mobile tip as it crept past the larynx. I watched the progress through my eye-piece and saw the pale membrane that was the gullet extending far away in front of me like an underground railway tunnel. Suddenly we entered a zone where the walls were ugly and red, pitted with ulcers – it was the bottom of the gullet in the inflamed condition known as oesophagitis. Advancing the endoscope now needed more effort; the tip was pressing into the muscular cardia, the valve at the opening of the stomach. Foamy brown liquid washed against the viewing lens and the control box hummed as David sprayed it away. The resistance to the onward journey of the tube ceased immediately we broke through into the interior of the stomach. David quickly inflated it with air and began to revolve the tip of the scope so that we could inspect its surroundings.

It was a horrific, almost surrealistic sight. Staring through my eye-piece, I became a pot-holer standing for the first time in a great crimson-walled grotto. Roof, walls, floor – everything was a bright and glistening red. From the ceiling dripped beads of blood that splashed into shallow pools of dark liquid, as it were around my feet. I had descended into one of Hieronymus Bosch's visions of Hell!

Approaching the wall at one point, I saw that it was pitted where patches of the lining had crumbled away. Our searchlight beam picked out another corroded area, then another; the walls were covered with ragged ulcers. No sign of food remains lay in the cavern. In the distance we could distinguish the exit at the pyloric valve, a portal that was also grotesquely puffy and inflamed. David angled the tip so that it touched, oh so gently, one of the walls. The wall at once began to bleed at the point of contact. The membrane was in a frighteningly delicate state. I heard the hissing as David pumped in more air.

'Come on, let's go through into the duodenum,' I said and, two intrepid cavers, we forged on with our eyes as the endoscope wormed its way through the door into the first part of the intestine. Once we had crossed the threshold of the pylorus things looked much better. The crimson decor instantly gave way to one of orange-tinged pink and the tunnel walls were firm and sound.

'Everything looks gradely in here,' said David, who was gazing at virtually the same 'underground' scenery that he'd surveyed less than eighteen hours previously in the lady in the Lancaster hospital.

'Let's go back and photograph all the stomach and oesophagus,' I replied, 'and take specimens of the wall and gastric juices.'

Chang-Chang, it was clear, had severe and acute ulceration of the stomach. The sooner we got the hell out of there and began treatment, the better. We set about collecting our samples – speleologists gathering fragments of stalagmites and rock-fall – and after ten minutes withdrew the endoscope.

To my delight, Chang-Chang was still breathing strongly and beginning to move his tongue, a sign of coming round. I gave him some injections of anabolic hormone to encourage tissue-healing and of pain-relieving analgesic and then we carried him back to his sleeping quarters and stood watching. My delight turned sour some five minutes later when his muscles began to quiver in a most curious manner; it reminded me of what I'd seen in wolves given heavy doses of certain experimental anaesthetics. The tremors spread and I began to fear that they might be a sign of over-dosage and lead to convulsions. Should I try to suppress them with a little barbiturate? I opted to grit my teeth and do nothing for the present. When I got down on my knees and blew into Chang-Chang's ear, he flicked it. Good, but the quivering continued. Thirty minutes passed, during which I aged perhaps five years, and then the strange tremors ceased abruptly and the panda staggered to his feet and pulled himself up onto his sleeping shelf. Funny, mysterious old panda – what an odd way of coming round, but it looked as if we'd got away with the anaesthesia OK. This time, at least.

'So what do you think, Doctor?' asked Dr Celma, who had come into the panda house during the operation and stood silently watching.

'Gastric ulcers. Not quite middle-aged businessman's disease, but something like it.'

'And what can we do for that?'

Everyone knows that a giant panda's favourite food is supposed to be bamboo, although in China I'd learned that wild pandas will travel miles to break into a forest-worker's hut and snatch roast pig or chicken after getting a whiff of it on the wind. In Madrid Shao-Shao and Chang-Chang, like all the pandas in captivity, were supplied with choicest fresh bamboo each day after it had been well washed to remove any lingering traces of pesticide from the leaves. Pandas aren't refined eaters. They don't nibble at things delicately but rather scrunch and gobble, and one can see in normal panda droppings how imperfectly they chew their food. Sizeable chunks of hard bamboo stem travel through the alimentary canal undigested. Having seen with my own eyes what the softest of touches with the smooth rubber tip of the endoscope could do to Chang-Chang's stomach lining, I decided to recommend the unthinkable.

'Stop all bamboo for Chang-Chang at once,' I said. Everyone looked aghast. A giant panda without bamboo was like Winnie-the-Pooh deprived of honey or Falstaff condemned to a diet of Perrier water. 'Not a scrap of fibrous food must he have,' I insisted. 'Out come the carrots and apples. He's going onto the blandest of bland diets suitable for a human peptic ulcer sufferer.'

I sketched out the regime I wanted. A basis of Complan, the British complete invalid food, milk, baby cereal, rice pudding, honey and eggs. For medicine I decided on cimetidine, the wonder drug that had revolutionised the treatment of folk with stomach ulcers. Chang-Chang would receive two tablets crushed into his food three times a day. 'And give him small meals but often,' I instructed, 'so that the powerful stomach acid can't build up too much.' With any luck the cimetidine would anyway cut down the production of panda stomach acid as efficiently as it does in man, dolphins and sealions.

My injections had eased the stomach ache that Chang-Chang must have suffered, and when he'd slept off all the effects of the anaesthetic later the same day he looked around for a little grub. I began the drugs at once. He seemed to enjoy the nourishing if queer-looking pudding that was now to be his daily fare and resembled one of the unattractive 'economy' dishes that I'd been developing for the pet cook-book. There was much smacking of his lips when he'd sucked up the first dishful.

Chang-Chang recovered from his stomach ulcers as rapidly, comparatively, as he had surfaced from the anaesthetic. Following the operation he did not vomit even once more, and began to behave in normal manic-depressive panda fashion, sleeping for long hours, then frolicking on the grass like a teddy bear and then going off for another comfortable nap. His appetite was gargantuan and he cared not whether the Complan base was strawberry, chocolate, banana or plain flavoured – down it all went with a satisfying slurp. Because the invalid food wasn't readily available in Spain we set up a system for importing it in boxes of one gross assorted flavours, and to speed things up in the first few weeks were granted use of the diplomatic bag of the Spanish embassy in London.

Most satisfactory of all, Chang-Chang put on twenty kilos in weight and his coat became rich and glossy. By the time David Wild and I returned at the end of five weeks to repeat the operation of scanning his stomach, he was in the pink and very perky. The endoscope examination went exactly as before and although I adjusted my ratios of valium and ketamine, the troubling tremors reappeared during the recovery period.

What a difference now in the stomach! The Grand Guignol stage-set that had confronted us before was now transformed into an Aladdin's cave with healthy walls of glistening pink and pools and rivulets of limpid digestive juices that sparkled and gave off wraiths of pearly vapour. Search our hidden vault as we might, we couldn't find a single ulcer remaining. Only the bottom end of the gullet still retained some inflammation of its lining.

I continued Chang-Chang's rigid diet for many months, although as soon as we'd seen the healed stomach I allowed a small quantity of the youngest and softest of bamboo foliage to be added. Confounding the panda pundits' idea of what pandas prefer, Chang-Chang didn't seem to relish the plant any more and he hasn't changed that point of view to any extent ever since. He still gets a diet based more on Complan than on bamboo. He loves it and it likes him, so who are we to argue?

If ever you're in Madrid, make a point of paying your respects to Chang-Chang and his mate at the zoo in the Casa de Campo, and when you read the sign outside their house that tells you a little about giant pandas, including 'their favourite food is, of course, bamboo', give Chang-Chang a wink. You and he both know better. He has been known to wink back!